1 MONTH OF
FREE
READING

at

www.ForgottenBooks.com

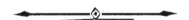

By purchasing this book you are eligible for one month membership to ForgottenBooks.com, giving you unlimited access to our entire collection of over 1,000,000 titles via our web site and mobile apps.

To claim your free month visit:

www.forgottenbooks.com/free1010017

ISBN 978-0-331-06727-9
PIBN 11010017

ESSAYS AND LECTURES

ON

MEDICAL SUBJECTS.

BY JOHN P. HARRISON, M. D.

PROFESSOR OF MATERIA MEDICA IN THE CINCINNATI COLLEGE.

PHILADELPHIA:

J. CRISSY, 4 MINOR STREET.

1835.

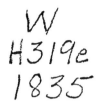

Printed by J. Crissy & G. Goodman, 4 Minor St.

PREFACE.

THE following Essays and Lectures on subjects of interest to Students of Medicine, are published from a conviction that the suggestions contained in them may prove of benefit to those, for whom they are intended. The conscientious, and modest, and aspiring student of medicine, occupies a trying and responsible position: he is often sorely agitated by an apprehension that, after the most sedulous and assiduous devotedness to a due preparation for the practice of medicine, he will prove deficient in practical skill—that however furnished with the acquisitions of elementary and doctrinal knowledge in his profession, he may nevertheless fail in that very point, in which it is all important for him to acquit himself well; in the resources of a sound, manly, discriminating judgment of diseases and of their remedies. This sense of afflicting doubt is replete with perplexity, and often depresses the sallies of his mind after high attainments, and robs his faculties of that elastic tone and bouyancy, which are essential to an animated prosecution of a complex scheme of science.

The Essay on Medical Experience, is intended to assist the student of medicine out of such embarrassment. No considerations are presented in it which can, in the remotest degree, be construed to imply that men can become skilful and enlightened practitioners of physic, without the most pains-taking devotement of their best powers to the study of this noble and useful branch of human knowledge. No. The working man must be found here, if any where; the science of medicine is the product of working men; and without industry, the most strenuous, directed in a proper path of protracted intellectual effort, no man, however gifted, can become a judicious and safe prescriber of remedial agents to his fellow men. Let the standard of medical literature be elevated by the urgent demand of the public for cultivated physicians, and then may we confidently expect that the profession will no longer be infested by such a host of ill educated, and ill prepared practitioners of the healing art.

The Lectures were delivered, as their respective title pages denote, in the city of Louisville, where the author resided, with the exception of a few years, nearly forty years.

With lively hopes that this little work may prove useful to the students of that science, which the author regards as the first of all mere human sciences in the wideness of its fruit of his labours with candour, and in the spirit which prompted to the publication.

PHILADELPHIA,

194 Arch St. Aug. 1835.

CONTENTS.

	PAGE
Essay on Medical Experience,	9
Address delivered before the Louisville Medical Society,	68
Lecture on the Influence of the Mind upon the Body,	84
Lecture on the Responsibilities of the Medical Profession,	112
Essay on the Diseases induced by Mercury,	125
A Statement of the circumstances connected with the sudden death of eight persons, who partook of Cold Custard, in Louisville, Ky.	181

MEDICAL EXPERIENCE.

THE illustrious restorer of modern science, in his Advancement of Learning, has given us an acute and just reflection in reference to the slow progress of medical science, which evinces his penetrating capacity of discrimination upon a subject so deeply interesting to the mind of every cultivated physician.

"Medicine," says he, "has been a science more professed than laboured, and yet more laboured than advanced; the labour having been, in my judgment, rather in a circle than in progression. For I find much iteration, but small addition."

Whoever, with a calm and enlightened spirit of observation, looks over the wide tract of medical history, will find ample materials for the judgment Bacon has passed upon our science. With here and there a light to direct the steps, we discover long intervals of dark and sterile ground.

There are two aspects in which medicine is to be contemplated.—One as an art, the other as a science. There are peculiar fallacies connected with each of these great leading divisions. And the fallacies of "too much learning" having more fascination about them, and being kept often from merited oblivion,

2

by the accompaniments of literary accomplishment,
deserve a more careful analysis at our hands, than the
fallacies of mere medical art, which from its ready
liability to degenerate into empirical pretension, meets
a quick exposure in the common sagacity of mankind.
And still human nature, true to itself under all circumstances and in every age, loves the luxury of delusion,
and most pertinaciously clings to exhibitions of the
wonderful, and often delights to yield itself up without
reserve, to an unlimited faith in the wisdom and superior skill of those who assume the ground of magisterial
dictation in matters pertaining to the knowledge and
cure of diseases.

Though delusion after delusion be exposed and perish, like images traced in sand by the sea-shore, which
the next wave obliterates, yet the spirit of delusion,
the love of deception, perish not, become not weary
with the progress of years, with the experience of time.
One form of error rises, is received with favour, eulogized as the messenger of great good to man, endures
for a season, till another one arises to supplant its older
rival, and like it, flourish in brief existence, then fades
away and is forgotten.

The science, as well as art of medicine, to the eye
of the philosophical beholder, resembles Virgil's mystical tree at the mouth of Avernus, thickly covered
with visionary leaves, and on every leaf a dream. But
it is a great and useful art, a noble and elevated science,
well deserving of the highest appreciation, and most
exalted esteem. For however obscured by error, and
perverted by quackery, the art of healing is the source
of many blessings to man. And as a science, medi-

cine is of liberal bearing, and full of intellectual greatness; having for its object the expansion of the human
mind on some of the most interesting topics that can
invite investigation. Man, in his physical frame, in
the organic structure, and physiological laws of that
frame,—in his capacities of thought and emotion, and
the inscrutable connexion of these divine capacities
with his physical frame,—in the diseases, so various
and numerous, which afflict his body and mind,—the
remedies which a sound experience has authenticated
as most proper to remove those diseases,—and the collateral and auxiliary sciences, which pour in their contributions of aid, of light, of power, into the storehouse
of this great and noble science.—All these attest the
dignity, and effectively proclaim the high and useful
bearing of medicine on the well-being of mankind.

Medicine may be correctly designated a scientific
art. For as art is the application of knowledge to a
practical end, and is empirical if acquired by expe-
rieuce alone, yet if that accumulated experience be
reasoned upon, and reduced to general principles, it
assumes a higher character, and thus constituted, becomes a scientific art.

The art of medicine is exclusively grounded in empirical experience, and is anterior in existence to any
deductions or general principles, which go to make the
science of medicine. Without this experience, medicine must ever remain a visionary and delusive theory,
and destitute of the inductive plan, of deducing general
principles from the data afforded by observation, it
would be a degraded and abject pursuit, lost in the
mysteries and technicalities of a mechanical occupa-

tion. It is the inherent tendency of the art of medicine, unaccompanied by the liberalizing and quickening energy of the science, to bury itself in concealed processes, to work in mystery, and attain its ends by short cuts, and often by "indirect crooked ways:" So that a due proportion of both of these elements, or main constituents, are absolutely essential toward the formation of a sound, authentic, enlightened experience in medicine.

In the whole compass of our language, there is scarce a word of greater latitudinarian construction, and of more indefinite import, than the word experience. And this holds with peculiar emphasis, as regards the daily application of the term to medicine. In no branch of human knowledge is there a more frequent employment of the word experience, than in medical science. To experience, a confident appeal is ever made by each party in a controversy concerning the curative efficacy of any particular remedy, or plan of treatment, to be adopted to remove an attack of sickness. The public in their excessive appreciation of the value of experience in our profession, deem no opinions wise, or ways of managing disease safe, but such as have upon them the broad impress and superscription of experience. Not knowing that error finds its safest lodgment in the intrenchments of a false experience,— that truth often has to combat on the open plain, unprotected by authority, and uncheered by the voice of acclaim, so readily bestowed on experience.

Experience, it is often averred by those who love to dogmatize on the narrow views they have derived from their own circumscribed opportunities of observation, and experience alone, must be our guide in arriving at just conclusions concerning the causes, nature and cure of diseases. But whilst such advocates of experience so confidently and pertinaciously insist on its exclusive authority in medicine, they seem unable to point out the boundary between experience and routine, and are incapable of attaching any comprehensive and generous intellectual appreciation to a term which appears to convey some talismanic power to their minds.

It has been an unfortunate thing for the progress of the mind in its career of improvement, that language has been so frequently perverted from its high function, as the just interpreter of thought, so as to become the shibboleth of prejudice, or the adopted watch-word of hereditary error. In its legitimate scope of agency, language is more than the interpreter of thought; it is embodied mind; it is tangible ideas; it is intellect made visible. But in order to accomplish these exalted purposes language must be employed with a constant and strict reference to its precise and determinate import. Ambiguity and imprecision should be banished from the language of every cultivated man, who wishes to impart his thoughts with force, perspicuity and certainty. Especially, in all discussions on physical phenomena, and in the explication of the laws which govern the material world, should all vagueness and indefiniteness of expression be excluded.

Medicine is a physical science, dependent for its successful cultivation on the same methods as other physical sciences. In medicine, the inductive philosophy has achieved some of its noblest trophies. In the several branches of anatomy, of physiology, of pharmacy, of therapeutics, instructed skill, patient observation, and accurate deduction have been the means by which physicians have been enabled to read nature in her operations, to compel her to give up her secrets to the expostulations of her ministers, and to answer the persevering interrogatories of her worshippers. Let poetry in her flights to the highest heaven of invention, deal in words which impart no definite conceptions to the mind, for it is amidst the grandeur of her sketches that she presents to the imagination glimpses of high objects, in a language too indefinite to provoke, and too sublime to allow the scrutiny of reason. But let the terms of medicine be well defined; let the language of physicians be the direct interpretation of the precise ideas existing in their minds; and let the nomenclature of our science be divested of all that cast of expression which, from its ambiguity, has so much retarded the human mind in the road of discovery.

The science of medicine owes much to experience, but it is an experience at once discriminative and profound. The collected light of ages beams around her path. To the assiduous and enlightened cultivators of our art from the days of Hippocrates to the present age of the world, we are indebted for that fund of facts and rational deductions which go to constitute the science of curing diseases. No one individual, in this age, should arrogate to himself an original experience, completely independent of the past experience of the medical world. Indeed, the most skilful in our art pretend to nothing more than a judicious combination of the experience of the past with their own observations—an application of that knowledge derived from erudition with that acquired by personal inspection, and a careful analysis of the opinions of their predecessors, so as to build upon it a manly and self-sustained judgment which shall enable them to disentangle the perplexities of disease, and to send a discriminating eye over all those details of medical practice which are so apt to embarrass and confuse weak minds.

Each physician must go through a discipline in the school of knowledge; each one has to advance from ignorance to wisdom by slow and measured steps; no man can, per saltum, reach the pinnacle of medical science; he might as well attempt to construct a dome without foundation. All valuable acquisition is the fruit of toil.

Dii laboribus omnia vendunt. Acquisitions collected with labour, are to be carefully preserved, and judiciously arranged. Out of this store, which a zeal for improvement, and a just ambition of distinction, have urged the individual to accumulate, he produces the treasures of mental riches. But without a correct conception of the great ends of our investigation—without a rational view of what we intend to accomplish, how shall we ever profit by the opportunities afforded for personal experience?

The subjects of medical knowledge are so varied—they lie scattered over such a vast field of inquiry, and are of such difficult investigation, that none but a mind disciplined by previous habits of study, and well-grounded in those elementary truths which prepare it for fruitful labour, can surmount the obstacles which hinder its advancement in the road of medical science. A perception of analogy and relation lies at the founda-

tion of all our intellectual attainments. It is, this which
constitutes the mental process by which we compare,
reason and judge.   Now, if our minds have never been
imbued with the best methods of exercising this per-
ceptive faculty; if the objects upon which it should be
exercised are not made familiar by a previous frequent
reference to the opinions entertained by others on the
points we intend to investigate, how shall we ever be
able to make a proper discrimination of the analogies
and relations—the contrarieties and resemblances, existing in the subjects offered to our examination.   By
learning to measure our strength before we rush into
the arena we shall be surer of success in the contest
which awaits us.   We must regulate the action and
measure of our faculties by a careful training, and thus
we prevent them being wasted in unproductive and
abortive efforts.   To this end choice and unity of purpose, as well as perseverance and method, are required.
We must, by our choice, determine what shall be the
subject for our investigation, and by a unity of purpose
economize our faculties, and increase their strength by
concentrating them.

Some physicians, feeling an incapacity for scientific
investigation, go on to amass a chaos of insulated facts
which they dignify by the term experience.   But it is
by cautious theory that experience can be perfected.
Between theory and experience, understood according
to their true meaning, there is neither contrast nor
opposition.   Who are the men that have given to medicine its chief glory as an intellectual pursuit?   They
are men who inferred general principles from a saga-
cious comparison of a great variety of phenomena.   And

this exercise of the reasoning faculties on the subjects of medicine is true theory. A correct experience, within its proper limitation, is nothing more than the handmaid of theory. Between an experience, enlightened and guided by theory, and an experience, gross and undistinguishing, there is the same difference as there is between the philosophy of Newton, and the matter-of-fact man that labours in the manufactory where the instruments are prepared by which the heavenly bodies are seen. To the first belong penetration, analysis and judgment—to the second there attaches only a blind routine which supersedes the exercise of the rational faculties.

The science of medicine in its legitimate spirit of candour, of liberality, and of the love of truth, seeks for an open and generous field, upon which it may exercise its powers, and display the rich fruits of its acquisitions. In accordance with the beautiful remark of the great master of the inductive philosophy, "it is an interpretation of nature"—its elements are simple, but its applications endless—and it binds together by a prolific principle of philosophy the scattered materials of our otherwise rude and shapeless art. Always partaking of the spirit of the age in which it may be cultivated, the science of medicine is indebted to the stirring genius of modern times, for its richest gifts, and most excellent accessions. Prompted to effort, and guided in the effort it makes, by the spirit of a true interpretation of nature, which a just consideration of the faculties of the human mind has imparted, it looks abroad, out from the narrow enclosure of personal experience, to the wide and fertile domains of a culti

vated science, as that science exists among the profession in all parts of the civilized world. And whilst
each physician must employ, most assiduously, the
powers of his own mind to discover what is truth in
the science of medicine, still he must not neglect to
advert to other minds, in order to derive from them
that light which his own limited experience, alone, will
never confer.

The inquiring, and conscientious, and aspiring physician, in imitation of our great countryman Rush, whose
whole life was one entire consecration of his ardent and
capacious mind, to the study of that science he so pas-
sionately loved, and so eloquently enforced, will, with
persevering toil strive, by consecutive investigation, to
attain a higher degree of knowledge, and adjust with
greater accuracy his attainments, each day of his professional life.

1 shall endeavour in the further discussion of the sub-
jcet, in as brief a manner as possible, to point out
the sources of false medical experience, and enumerate
some of the many follies which it has engendered and
propagated; and in the next place notice the best
methods of acquiring a true medical experience, and
expatiate a little on the immense benefits to be derived
from such a source of knowledge.

1. *False Medical Experience.* —The principal
sources of the many "false facts" by which every
department of human knowledge is more or less
vitiated are the following. 1. Superstition. 2. Credulity. 3. Fallacy of testimony. 4. Ambiguity of
language. 5. False theory.

It is difficult to bring errors into any regular classifi.

cation. Truth is one and the same, but error puts on infinite and ever-varying aspects: from its essential nature it appears to have no limits and no end. But the limits it has not in itself, it has in the nature of the objects about which it is conversant, and from the con-stitution of the mind. In medicine there are a certain number of outlets by which the mind forsakes the straight way of truth. These have been indicated by several respectable writers, such as Zimmerman in his work on Experience in Physic, Paris in his Pharma-cologia, and Sir Gilbert Blane in his Medical logic. I have selected from them the principal sources of false medical experience, and shall as succinctly as possible point them out.

1. *Superstition.*—Ignorance is the foodful nurse of that belief which reposes in security on the extraordi-nary and supernatural agency of remedies in them-selves inert and ineffective. In the twilight of mind, objects assume an adventitious appearance. Fancy peoples the vacuity of ignorance with endless delusions. Instead of penetrating the true causes of phenomena, and tracing out the harmony which marks the bene-ficent arrangements of nature, the mind infected with superstition goes out in eager quest of strange and ano-malous fortuities, and is ceaselessly employed in con-juring up phantoms, which terrify and rule the soul.

The history of all human science bears mournful evidences on its ample page, of the corrupting influence of superstition. Even among the Greeks those who first attempted to assign the natural causes of thunder and lightning were condemned as the enemies of the gods. The fate of Galileo is familiar to all. Medicine

has been deeply tinctured with a reliance on superstitious remedies.   Among savage tribes of mankind, the
whole art of curing disease consists in the practice of
ridiculous, disgusting mummeries.   Among the Chilian
Indians the only mode of relieving the sick is by
blowing round their beds, so that if a doctor can blow
well, he is sure to obtain a good business.   But even
philosophers have manifested superstition in matters
relating to the cure of diseases.   Boyle asserts, that he
saw a sympathetic powder effect a speedy restoration
to health, and he places great reliance on the thigh
bone of an executed criminal for the cure of dysentery.
The great mind of Lord Bacon was darkened by a
superstitious belief in charms and amulets.   An extraordinary virtue was attached by Soranus to the honey
that was produced by bees that lived near the tomb of
Hippocrates.   Among the Druids of Gaul and Britain,
who were both priests and physicians, the misletoe,
gathered with a gold knife, when the moon was six
days old, and consecrated by incantations, was esteemed
an infallible antidote to poisons, and a preventive of
sterility.   Galen is considered as the author of the anodyne necklace, so long famous among the great and
little vulgar of England.   He asserts that if threads are
tied about the neck of a viper so as to suffocate it, and
afterwards tied around a patient's neck, they will cure
all kinds of tumours arising on it.   The royal touch of
England, and the use of amulets and charms sprang
from the same source.

The three most intense of human predilections considering man as an intellectual, social, and physical
being, are the main avenues through which tyranny

has made its most successful approaches, in rude states of society. These are, the strong desire man feels for ne preservation of life, the irrepressible aspirings of his nature towards religious emotion, and his earnest want for some kind of polity. In ignorant and rude conditions of society there is often a union of the functions of the physician, priest and chief, in one individual. We need not, however, draw our illustrations in the present instance from barbarous tribes, for the celebrated Prince Hohenlohe, perhaps still alive, will furnish a most apposite example of such a species of folly.

Alexander Leopold Hohenlohe, a Hungarian prince, whose father was disqualified for government by mental derangement, and whose mother was of an ardent temperament, and of fervid zeal for her religion, began in 1815 to manifest his talents for preaching agreeably to his fond mother's hopes and entreaties. "After having received the papal permission to consecrate three thousand rosaries, crucifixes, &c. at once, he left Rome and went to Germany, where he was considered by his colleagues as devoted to Jesuitism, and an enemy to knowledge." Martin Michel, in Baden, a worker of miraculous cures, through the power of faith, and the efficacy of prayer, assured the Prince, that the faith and prayers of a prince, were of much greater prevalence and potency to effect miraculous cures than were those of a common peasant, such as Michel was. The imagination of the fanatic prince was fired at once, and he soon proceeded to put into execution Michel's plan of healing the halt, the blind, the impotent, and the insane. A princess, Matilda, of Schwartzenburg, who had distortion of the spine, was made to walk, through the agency of the princely priest and doctor, aided by Michel, his guide, encourager and friend. The prince soon, however, commenced operations on his own responsibility and prayers, and multitudes eagerly crowded around his path. This spiritual phy-sician's fame soon diffused itself over Germany, the country of the ideal, and reached even England and America. His enthusiastic admirers published many, in their opinion at least, veritable cases of terrible dis-ease, which they solemnly averred were cured by this great apostle of delusion. He could not succeed in his cases in the hospitals of Würtzburg and Bamberg, and a prince of Hiedburghausen, who laboured under an affection of the eyes, in consequence of discontinuing all medical applications, and relying on this spiritual doctor, found his eyes soon get much worse. Still the confidence of Hohenlohe was, so great, and his pre-sumption so overweening, that in 1821, he solicited the Pope's attention to his miraculous endowment, but Pius VII, intimated his will to be, that the process should not be designated a miracle, but *priestly prayer for healing.*

After Hohenlohe's failure upon the prince, with diseased eyes, he declared himself exhausted, and was unwilling to be seen by the health police whilst in the act of performing his cures. Of late, he works at a distance, and the newspapers, and some of the medical periodicals, have given us accounts of the reputed miracles performed by his highness, or excellency, in France, England, Scotland, Ireland and the United States. His mode of late, is to direct the afflicted person, making application for cure to him, to pray at certain times of the day, cotemporaneously with him. self. It has been objected to these simultaneous prayers by some caviling spirits, that a prayer at 8 o'clock, in Hungary, has been ended before that of .8 o'clock, at Marseilles begins; but to this objection, urged by the sceptic, one irrefutable reply is enough, it is all miracle, or all superstition—from alpha to omega—and admits no investigation, but demands a simple, unquestioning faith, too facile for doubt, and too submissive for reply.*

The above furnishes a melancholy proof of the perverted application of that scheme of human illumination, which Christianity furnishes, and is a signal verification of a remark already made, that mankind love the luxury of delusion, and seek its gratification in the most exhorbitant exhibitions of folly.

2. *Credulity.*—This vice of the mind is nearly allied to superstition; ignorance is the mother of both. But though derived from the same parent, they differ 'in some essential features. Credulity gives credence to propositions unsustained by sufficient data. The credulous man believes extravagant accounts of the virtues of medicines, perhaps in themselves potent, but not possessed of all the virtues ascribed to them. Novelty spreads a bewildering gloss on remedies, to the eye of him who has not a sufficient maturity of judgment to resist its fascinations. A warm and animated zeal for any cause, unless that zeal is chastened and regulated by a severe discipline of judgment, is sure to mislead

---

* Encyclop. Americana: article, Hohenlohe.

the mind. Quod volumus, facile credimus, is as true
in medicine as in the ordinary pursuits of life. ' Our
science is filled with convincing illustrations of this
position. The discoverer of every new remedy asserts
that he finds in it an epitome of the whole *materia
medica.* The metallic tractors of Perkins, the animal
magnetism of Mesmer, the elixir of life of Paracelsus,
the alkahest of Van Helmont, and the panaceas and
catholicons of the present day, all have derived their
source from fraud operating on credulity. Even where
no sordid considerations influence the propagator of a
revived, or newly discovered remedy, the ardent enthusiasm of the experimenter urges him to great extravagance in the commendations he bestows on it. Baron
Storck greatly overrated the remedial power of the
Narcotics upon which he made so many experiments.
There is no prominent remedy in our catalogue of
agents for the removal of disease, but what has been at
one time surrounded by a mist of panegyric. And how
many inert substances have been eulogized, that are
now quietly slumbering in the tomb of forgetfulness!
Opium, digitalis, mercury, antimony, and the bark are
the most effective weapons of medicine. Each of these
have been injured in their legitimate character, as
medicinal substances, by the indiscriminate encomiums
lavished upon them. The most enlightened physicians
now agree with the illustrious Sydenham, "that the
practice of physic chiefly consists in being able to discover the true curative indications and not medicines
to answer them; and those that have overlooked this
point have taught empirics to imitate physicians."

Credulity delights in going in constant search of anomalies and novelties. When a new remedy is suggested for some incurable malady, such as Prussic acid for tubercular consumptions, or scutellaria for hydrophobia, the credulous minded physician does neither hesitate, nor suspend his judgment, but rushes to a precipitate conclusion, and upon some very inaccurately observed isolated case proclaims his unlimited confidence in the article. It is in the rank soil of credulity that quackery flourishes, and sends forth its luxuriant branches.

The *Eau Medicinale d'Husson* not many years since was implicitly relied on for the cure of gout, and the case of Sir Joseph Banks was quoted in its favour. What now is the just opinion attached to that nostrum by the most learned men of our profession ? Let any one read what the profound Parry says about it, and he will at once be convinced of the injurious agency of the remedy, in preventing regular paroxysms of a constitutional disease, and thus exposing the patient to the imminent peril of apoplexy, or palsy, or some other severe attack of disease.

The doctrine of Signatures in the choice of remedies sprung from the same source, an excessive credulity. Fox's lungs were given to cure asthma, because the animal was capable of running long before he became exhausted. Turmeric, from its yellow colour, was administered as a sure cure for jaundice.

Under the head of credulity most appropriately, perhaps, are to be included the reveries and figments of Hahnemann's subtle but prolific brain. Endowed to a degree far beyond the common rate of even Germanic ideality, and metaphysical vapouring, the author of the system of Homæopathy, has challenged human credulity to the utmost, and put to test the strength of man's addictedness to abandon his mind to the wildest wanderings of hypothesis: if the hypothesis is enforced by confident appeals to testimony, and a determined hostility towards all established views. Mixing up with the crudest modes of explaining the action of remedies, much parade of learning and professions of philanthropy, the abettors of this system, most emphatically denounce and vilify all the generally established modes of considering, and of treating, disease. The captivating blandishments of infallibility and impeccability are, of course, the supreme features of homæopathism. It is the wisest, safest, best, and most sure mode of treating all human maladies. All other plans of conducting the treatment of disease are, in comparison to the homæopathic, but mere clumsy artifices of medical skill, mere potent engines of perpetuating morbid action, and of perpetrating death. Hahnemann, like another Bacon, has promulgated his organon, the leading doctrinal peculiarity of which is, *similia, similibus curantur,* in accordance with which to cure a disease, you must administer medicines that will excite symptoms similar to the disease—and thence is derived the name of the system, homæopathy, or as it is sometimes written homoopathy—from the Greek words, ὅμοιον alike, and παδος disease.

Experience is, with exceeding vehemence, appealed to by the homæopathists as the test and supporter of their wise, and safe and certain plan of eradicating morbid action from the system. And their experience—it is a distinct and peculiar experience—assures them that chamomile flowers excite 1480 symptoms—iron produces 228—bark 469—platinum 402—and elder-flowers 116!! A drop of the spirituous tincture of sarsaparilla is a strong dose, and a seven-millionth part of a grain of *cucumis colocynthis* acts very often with too much potency!*

Dr. Rau, another metaphysical genius of the land of the indefinite and abstract, has given the following among other cases to prove the verity of the homæopathic therapeutics. A feeble attenuated woman, sixty-two years old, had suffered from repeated attacks of pneumonia and difficulty of breathing; and during an acute attack of fever, pain in the side, frequent cough, &c., Dr. Rau gave her the billionth part of a drop of the expressed juice of aconite, mixed with a drachm of water. Very soon a thilling sensation spread over her frame—a perspiration came on—the pain, fever, cough, all disappeared; and after a sound night's repose, she awoke in renovated existence, and seizing the doctor by the hand, when he visited her, she exclaimed with rapture that she was well! In a patient affected with a frightful dropsy, accompanied by great prostration of strength, coldness of the whole body, and inability to discharge more than a few drops of urine, a single very minute dose of the tincture of black hellebore, relieved all the symptoms in a few days.†

Reason and facts are of no avail in a warfare of disputation with such medical mystics. Men, whose senses are steeped in the most absurd credulity, and

---

* See Edin. Med. and Surg. Journal, vol. 28, p. 61.

† Amer. Journal of Med. Science, for Feb. 1831.

whose judgments are abandoned to the wildest dreams
of folly. We must deliver them over to the same
category of imaginative and rapt enthusiasm, as that
which possessed the seething brains of Emmanuel Swe-
denborg, who talked familiarly with angels and devils,
and had revelations and visions as divine as the second
sight in Scotland. Should the reader wish to read a
most elaborate refutation of homæopathy, let him, with
German patience, sit down to Dr. Leo-Wolf's book,
entitled, Remarks on the Abracadabra of the Nineteenth
Century; or on Dr. Samuel Hahnemann's Homæopa-
thie Medicine. The following passage from this vigorous assailant of the homæopathic delusion, is evinsive
of a fond addictness to other reveries about as well
founded as those of Hahnemann.

"Thus animal magnetism"—the author is giving an
illustration of the discoveries of German medical men;
and seriously adduces animal magnetism as a proper
topic of eulogy!—"Thus" says he, "animal magnetism, first mentioned about three centuries ago by Paracelsus, a German, and introduced as a remedy about
sixty years since, by Mesmer, also a German, remained
almost unnoticed by all other nations, the French
excepted, although many professional men in Germany
still apply this great agent as a remedy which, here-
after, will be more generally appreciated, when likewise divested of the mystery which fancy and credulity
have so long combined with it." And when that
divesture takes place, what will be left of animal magnetism? Take away the fancy and credulity which
were at work in its creation, and are now so operative
in keeping it alive, and it will share the fate of its great

progenitor, Paracelsus Theophrastus Bombastus de Hohenheim—the celebrated empiric and alchemist—or that of its reviver, the great magnetizer, whose delusions our illustrious Franklin aided in detecting and exposing. And Paracelsus and Mesmer were Germans! happy land to give birth to a pair of such transcendental and sublime sons of fancy and folly—of visions and vanities!

3. *Fallacy of Testimony.*—It was the remark of a celebrated teacher of medicine, that there are in our science more false facts than false theories. Paradoxical as this may seem, its truth is established by the most comprehensive and accurate observations which can be made on the wide field of practical medicine. Wherever we turn our eyes, whatever part of the field we may contemplate, there rises before us a thick cloud of false facts. There is no department of our art so overrun with the fruits of false experience as the materia medica. The best and most approved authorities of that branch of medicine have made this statement. Whence originates this lamentable state of things ? Why is it that this valuable department of our science should abound in such uncertainties, and be oppressed by such a load of useless remedies? It is clear that in order to ascertain with precision the veritable operation of any remedy, three conditions are required. 1st. Whether the patient is really afflicted with the disease for the cure of which the remedy is to be administered. 2nd. After the remedy is given, whether or not the patient is cured at all; and 3d. whether, if cured, it was the remedy which cured him, or he got well in despite of it.

The great importance of Sydenham's remark is now more distinctly perceived. Unless the physician under-stands the nature of the disease and from that. know-ledge gathers the indications of cure, of what avail is it that he has a long catalogue of medicines to administer? Here the paramount consequence of a true theory reveals itself. It is upon the well established basis of a correct pathology that the thiumphs of our science are achieved. Here charlatanry stands rebuked, by the well sustained principles of scientific investigation; here it "loses, discountenanced, and into folly turns." Very frequently, reputed cures are discovered to be only a partial suspension of the onward career of a malady: The dominant control exercised by imagina-tion over the excitable hopes of a patient suffering under some chronic affection operates a very great influence on the body. It is in this way that the supposititious cures of Mesmer and Perkins were accomplished. It is in this manner that charms and amulets have sometimes suspended the progress of a fatal disease. In many instances of this kind the patient has no real disease, but is under the dominion of a gloomy and fantastic fancy. The case of stone, supposed at the time to have been cured by Mrs. Stephen's remedy, for which Par-liament liberally rewarded her, is in point. In that instance we have a verification of the fallacy of medical testimony. The patient was examined by medical men of the highest reputation, and upon their declara-tion of his being cured, the reward was granted. But the man still laboured under the stone, only it was con-cealed from detection by the sound, by its being in-vested in a sac of the bladder. The reputation of other nostrums has been reared on a similar perishable foundation. The fallacy of testimony is forcibly illustrated in - the asseverations of some of the older writers, respecting the presence of globular mercury in the bones. The solemn march of the germs of the future animal in the semen of a ram, which drew forth such wonderment from Boerhaave, stands on the same grounds; and so the contagiousness of bilious remittent and yellow fever, is advocated by those who place too much credence in fallacious evidence. Fordyce attempts to prove that common remittent fever is contagions, and the advocates of the contagiousness of yellow fever are found in the highest ranks of the profession. Coincidence is taken for causation—the *post hoc* occupies the place of the *propter hoc* on such occasions. In consequence of that prevailing link of sympathy which binds together men in society, there spreads at times a sort of universal assent to any, however extravagant, statement. Thus the mind of each one seems predisposed to admit, without due examination, the slightest proof as corroborative of the remedial efficacy of any new article of the materia medica. Physicians partake of this feature of mind with other men. They too are easily satisfied with the testimony afforded in substantiation of the virtues of a novel remedy. Hence it is that so many in our profession stand ready to

" Catch, e'er she fall, the Cynthia of the minute."

Hence it is that medicine seems more like a magic lantern, where the scene is perpetually shifting, than like the sober light of the great orb of day.

Perhaps a more conspicuous instance could not be

adduced to show the utter incompetency of a limited
personal experience to furnish a fair attestation to the
real value of a medicine, than the history of digitalis
affords. Dr. Beddoes at one time thought that in this
remedy he had a sure and safe means of arresting pulmonary consumption. But the experience of the profession generally, has deprived the plant of those extraordinary powers so blindly attributed to it, as regards
the cure of phthisis.

It were a task of immense labour to advert, by special enumeration, to all the numerous cases of such
fallacy, as that arising from extravagant views of the
medical properties of the various agents, which from
age to age, and from year to year, have received the
unsparing and undistinguishing eulogies of physicians.
And not contented to expatiate on the virtues of medicines which the ingenuous dealer in drugs kept, appropriately labeled, in his shop, the most accomplished
physicians have at times departed from the employment of the remedies known to the profession, or
recommended by men of scientific candour, and too
enthusiastically attached themselves to the use, and too
eagerly recommended remedial agents, whose composition was a secret, and the authors and vendors of
which, knew nothing of the just principles of medical
science.

The splendour which at one time surrounded the
reputation of Swaim's Panacea, was derived from the
dazzling brilliancy of that light which several of the
luminaries of our American medicine threw around it.
With precipitate and onward haste, some of our most
enlightened physicians were found swelling the loud

chorus of praise which was sounding forth the many virtues and transcendent excellencies of this nostrum. Certificates, signed by several of the most eminent medical men of the country, quickly found their way into the newspapers, and were by them rapidly disseminated through the Union.

A regular graduate of our oldest medical school, became agent for Swaim, and went on a mission to England to vend the nostrum to our transatlantic brethren. But John Bull was not quite so gullible as brother Jonathan in this matter, and the mission proved abortive. That the reader may have the benefit of higher authority than the writer of this essay, I will copy a page or two from the "First Report of the Committee of the Philadelphia Medical Society, on Quack Medicines, read on the 15th December, 1827, and ordered to be published by the Society."

"Dr. Chapman acknowledges having 'overrated the value of the Panacea of Swaim,' and 'for a long period' he has 'entirely ceased to prescribe it'—says he has in possession not a few cases, which, if desired, are at the committee's service, and 'eminently calculated to alarm the public on this subject.' September 29th, 1827.

"Dr. Gibson says, he has found the Panacea succeed in cases of secondary syphilis, and fail in others; and adds, 'I have never found the remedy of any service in scrofula. In several cases which came under my notice, ptyalism has followed the use of it.' October 25th, 1827."

Dr. Dewees' experience of this article having been found useful, is limited to "four, or, at most, five

4

cases;" whereas his own practice, in which he has prescribed it several times, does not, he acknowledges, furnish a single case of any decided advantage following its use. October 26th, 1827. Dr. Dewees does not state the evidence on which he gave his certificate to Swaim; but, it is believed, that not even half of the few favourable results now alluded to, had then come under his own personal observation."

"Dr. Parke's statement, in his letter of September 28th, 1827, is, that he witnessed the case of Tregomain in the Pennsylvania Hospital; who, after being subjected to various methods of treatment, was finally cured by the somewhat prolonged use of Swaim's Panacea. The disease was a very obstinate malignant ulcer on her hand. It may be well to remark, that Dr. Parke's certificate in favour of the nostrum, was furnished on the strength of this *single case*. It would be a subject of curious inquiry, to ascertain the probable number of certificates to which the practice in a large hospital would give rise, in the course of a single year, if the cure of every case of a somewhat protracted disease were to lay claim to such notices. The valuable Hospital Reports, published from time to time, in various cities, would then give place to hospital *certificates*, with an effect on the march of medical improvement, of too painful a nature to be contemplated." Dr. Parke goes on to speak of two ladies from southern States, the melancholy nature and result of which, so totally different from the tenor of his letter, will be laid before the Society in a subsequent part of this report, in which it will also be seen that little, if any, credit can be attached to the Panacea as a remedial agent in Tregomain's case."

· "It seems then, from the testimony of those whose certificates in favour of Swaim's Panacea, have been so much relied on by the proprietor, and his friends and coadjutors, that nothing is adduced in them, calculated to inspire any confidence, whatever, in its use. On the contrary, Dr. Chapman's having long since ceased to prescribe it, and his pointing out cases of its alarming effects; Dr. Gibson's never having seen it succeed in scrofula; the constant failures, when Dr. Dewees has prescribed it, added to Dr. Parke's inexperience of its use, are all circumstances, well calculated to deter from recommending it."

"The committee, after a careful examination of the evidence, both written and verbal, submitted to them, respecting the sensible properties, presumed composition, and curative and deleterious effects on the animal economy, of Swaim's Panacea, are led to the following conclusions and opinions. The syrup, when free from any mercurial preparation, not only fails to exhibit virtues as a curative agent, superior to various compound decoctions and syrups of sarsaparilla, which have been administered in the regular practice of medicine for the last two hundred and fifty years, in the different stages of syphilis, and in chronic rheumatism and cutaneous complaints, but is inferior in efficacy to some of them, as well on account of the variableness of its composition, as from the occasional loss of the medical properties, and the adulteration of certain articles entering into it." p. 24.

It is a matter of deep regret to the committee, as they are well assured it has long been to the Society, that circumstances should render it necessary to enforce a position, the truth of which has always been admitted by thinking men in every profession, and which was received as an axiom among physicians. A hope, may now, however, be resonably entertained, that although the correctness of the general principle has not, as in former times, carried with it entire conviction, the direct specification of facts will, in future, produce unanimity of sentiment among medical men, notwithstanding the partial aberration into which some of them may, in a moment of misplaced good nature, have been betrayed. The time is now come, or more correctly speaking, the necessity is as urgent as ever, for a line of demarkation to be drawn between the advocates of empiricism, with all its unavoidably attendant train of evils, and the rightful members of a liberal profession, the friends of learning and of science. What physician, who retains the high conscientious feelings of his noble calling, will subject himself to the imputation of conniving with error for the wages of imposture; or, will be the eulogist of empirics and empiricism, console himself with the hard alternative of escaping judgment of corruption, at the expense of his understanding; even though an observing world should allow him the option of his sentence?" p. 26.

I cannot dismiss the consideration of this particular case—so pregnant with cogent proof of the fallacy of testimony, and so apposite in the lesson it should impart, of the imperative necessity of great intellectual caution in too readily rushing to premature conclusions, in reference to the powers of any remedy from a very limited personal trial of its curative efficacy,—without an expression of high regard for the sentiments, quoted above. And when it is remembered that such men as Horner, Harris, Klapp, Meigs and Bell, constituted the committee which made the report;—physicians whose high reputation in the profession, and honourable bearing, and courageous consistency in the discharge of the responsible duties of that profession, are known and recognized by the faculty throughout our country,—when such ornaments and firm pillars of medical science, attach their names to a publication, we have ample warrant of the justness of the opinions, the correctness of the statements, and the elevated medical morality, pervading its entire body. And a careful perusal of the Report most emphatically confirms the preconceptions, which a bare announcement of its authors would create. May the spirit of a vile, degrading, and ruinous charlatanry be rebuked by this Report, and may every cultivated and honest physician through society, maintain an impregnable position against the encroachments of quackery;—refusing, most resolutely and pertinaciously, any participation in its spoils, and making every effort, consistent with the purest ethics, to put down all the machinations of such imposture! To do this most effectively, every physician who regards his character and standing in the profession, should refuse consultation with any nostrum-vender, or pretender to secret remedies, and hold all such in low estimation, who do consult with such impostors.

4. *Ambiguity of Language* —This is an exuberant fountainhead of error in every species of intellectual inquiry. Accurate language subserves, in our profession, three important purposes. First, as an instru-

4 *

ment of intellectual analysis. Secondly, precision of expression affords a medium for distinctness of thought, like a clear atmosphere gives the eye the best opportunity of perceiving the exact outlines of bodies. Thirdly; accuracy of language is the only sure interpreter of perspicuous views; for imprecise and indefinite language is always the result of a clouded and confused comprehension of a subject. It would be well for every young man, who is preparing for the practice of medicine, to read over most carefully Locke's admirable chapter on the necessity for clear and accurate expression as the elucidation of truth. For says that great man, the want of a precise signification in words is the cause of very obscure and uncertain notions. There are two words of great currency in the profession which will afford an apposite illustration of the ambiguity of medical language. These words are *congestion* and *sympathy*. It is apparent that the words congestion and sympathy are generic; that they are similar to the word inflammation, which comprehends several species of diseased action. Whenever, therefore, such generic words are employed to convey ideas relative to a species, or a variety, they are misapplied. Thus, without pausing now to examine the correctness of the pathological views involved, when we read of congestion of the brain, or liver, or lungs, do we acquire from such indefinite language any exact and precise views of the condition of the affected organ? Such fashionable words do little in conveying accurate impressions to the reader's mind. Like general reflections they can never elucidate practical points in medicine. The writer must enter into detail, and do much

by circumstances. Nothing can elucidate but what is
pointed. Every remark must particularize and specify.
The eye may take in a large range, but the mind is
affected by inspection. We must descend from the
brow of a hill, and come down to certain spots and
objects. The science of medicine can never be much
benefited by such general, diffusive, and indefinite language as that employed by many writers. Thus when
they have designated a fever congestive, or when they
have ascribed the origin of a disease to sympathy, or
have traced all attacks of febrile affections to inflammation in the stomach, they seem to imagine that their
task is finished, and that they have completely satisfied
the reader as to the pathology of the disease. But
what precise views does he derive from such language?
The great advantage, to the writer at least, of such
language is, that it saves all further difficulty in his
description of a disease. But the reader is completely
beclouded in his apprehension of the pathological condition of the suffering organ, when he is told that it is
congested. What is congestion? he is ready to inquire.
This I will endeavour to answer before this discussion
closes.

5. *False Theory.*—It is a well established fact that
some of the most erroneous theories in medicine have
originated from men, who professed to despise theory.
And those men who are most addicted to expressions
of contempt against reasoning in medicine, are the
most disposed to indulge in crude speculation. And
the cause of this is obvious; it springs from too exclusive reliance on their own individual experience,
apart and independent of that accumulated wisdom of

ages to be found in books. " To think is to theorize,"
is a proposition not to be successfully controverted. So
deep in man's intellectual nature is laid that disposition
to account for phenomena, on which all philosophy is
built, that he cannot be induced to forego the gratification it affords, under any condition of his being. The
employment of reducing truth to its element, is one of
the most gratifying and useful occupations of the mind.

The luxuriant growth of our science, from the multitude of facts which have been collected by its assiduous
cultivators, demands that comprehensive and accurate
principles should be deduced from its many and insulated particulars. It is the object of correct theory to
reduce the multifarious appearances of disease to simplicity and order. In the present state of our science,
there is an imperative necessity for the exercise of an
inquisitive and powerful reason, to remodel and arrange
the facts that are already ascertained, and to trace up
the analogies which run through diseases to some general principles. Thus we shall be enabled to make a
discriminating survey of the miscellaneous variety of
particulars which are placed beneath our observation.
To frame a correct theory we must keep in mind the
remark of a distinguished medical teacher—"Medi-
cina neque agit in cadaver neque repugnante natura
aliquid proficit"—that medicine will neither act on a
dead body, nor will it act on a living body, in a way
contrary to the laws of the animal organization. It is
from an utter forgetfulness, or contempt, of this essential principle that the science has been infested by so
many chemical and mechanical theories. The humoral
pathology rested on a fallacious and shallow conception

of the laws of life. The nervous system, which constitutes the living being in contradistinction to the
organized dead mass of animal matter, was overlooked,
its structure was disregarded, and its laws unobserved.

But as the sun of medical science has ascended, the
mists which hung around the path of improvement are
disappearing. In exact proportion to the spread of
correct views on the anatomy and physiology of the
body has been the retreat of the humoral pathology.
Instead of physcians speaking in unintelligible language
of lentor, and alkalescency, of fermentation and concoc-
tion, and of virus floating in the blood, we hear of correct statements of symptoms, and of the actions going
on in the solids. What has humoralism ever done for
medicine?. It has retarded its march, it has shut up
the avenues to its successful cultivation, and deterio-
rated the genuine spirit of correct investigation.

To particularize. Scrofula was once attributed to a
vitiation, or depravity of the fluids, and the treatment
was empirical in accordance with such an erroneous
pathology. Since the renunciation of this erroneous
pathology, and the adoption of a correct view of the
disease as one of the solids, the treatment has been established on scientific principles. And so it has been
with gout, rheumatism, syphilis, small-pox and several
other affections.

Dr. Armstrong's popular doctrine of congestion is
founded on wrong views of anatomy and physiology,
and is therefore untenable. Indeed at page 288 of his
work on Typhus, under the head of common continued
fever, we have an admission that congestion and inflammation are the same. "The action of one artery,"

says he, "I have never known greater than that of another, and what we call increased action is, I suspect, merely increased accumulation; and what we call increased determination is, I also suspect, merely an increased volume of the vessels, arising from an impediment to the return of the blood from the quarter to which those vessels lead." And at page 159 of his Essay on Pulmonary Consumption he makes the same admission of the oneness or identity of congestion and inflammation. "It necessarily follows that when the energy of the heart and arteries is much diminished, that they cannot maintain the natural current of arterial blood, and of course a proportionate accumulation takes place in the veins; and this venous congestion appears to load and stimulate the capillaries of the arterial system by retarding the return of the blood through them." Four widely different pathological states of the system may be mistaken for congestion.

1st. Sympathetic derangement from worms; or ingesta in the alimentary canal; or from uterine irritation giving rise to hysteria.

2d. Constitutional irritation from surgical operations, loss of blood, or severe burns.

3d. Suffocated excitement, or such an intense degree of action as to overwhelm the powers of life. This often occurs in the yellow fever.

4th. Collapse of the powers of life in the last stage of fever. Dr. Potter, in his edition of Armstrong, admits that "the symptoms so formidable at the close of fevers are often nervous only, and the seeming congestion of as much importance as they are in hysteria."

The Broussaian pathology of fever is amenable to a

just objection an account of its generality. It is a recommendation to many minds, not disposed to scrutinize, that such pathological views involve no laborious process of thought, and demand no extensive examination. They are light and portable, easily transferred from the author's page to the reader's comprehension. The memory alone is exercised in their reception. To remember that every case of fever is nothing but congestion in the liver, or a gastro enteritis, is quite a compendious mode of arriving at a knowledge of the pathology of a class of diseases, whose history, nature and practice have tasked the mightiest intellects of our profession. And then the by-cut; the saving of thought; and the fallacious facility it gives to practice! The allurement held out by the simplicity of Brown's system enraptured, for a while, the medical world, especially the younger members of it. Dr. Rush's unity of disease rose with overpowering lustre above all other views of pathology, but it has long since fallen "like an exhalation in the night, to rise-no more," unless Broussais' gastro enteritis, or Armstrong's congestion, assume its guise, and limp after it in awkward imitation.

Without a correct knowledge of the laws which govern the animal economy, it is at once apparent to the discerning mind that medicine, as a science of just philosophy, can never attain either stability in its doctrines, or certainty in the means which it may suggest for the cure of disease.

No just and comprehensive views can be entertained of morbid action, by the physician who is ignorant of the physiological actions of the human structure. We

may safely infer, therefore, that the ancient doctrines
of the four elements, and of their corresponding temperaments, of the separate functions of the vegetative,
sentient and animal spirits, which were prevalent in
the schools of medicine from the time of Galen to the
middle of the seventeenth century—never could guide
to an enlightened analysis of the symptoms, and conduct to a just conception of the nature of either functional or structural disease.

The superstitious regard paid to antiquity, by some
learned, but feeble minds in our profession, is in sad
contrast to the animating spirit of improvement so dif-
fusively abroad in the general mass of every civilized
society. "Antiquity," says Bacon, "deserveth that
reverence that men should make a stand thereupon,
and discover what is the best way; but when the discovery is well taken, then to make progression. And
to speak truly, 'Antiquitas seculi, juventus mundi.'
These times are the ancient times, when the world is
ancient, and not those which we account ancient *ordine
retrogrado*, by a computation backward from ourselves."

To go to our ancient predecessors for a true pathology of disease, or the most successful mode of cure,
would be, to borrow a striking figure of Cabanis, to
imitate the two sons of Noah, who went backward to
cover their father's nakedness; thus manifesting their
filial piety, and at the same time evincing that the act
involved some degree of humiliation on their part.
Shall we attempt to follow the eclecticism of Boerhave,
and thus, instead of one error of our own origination,
amass together in a heterogeneous incorporation, the

fallacies and follies of the most opposite sects? He is designated as a very candid eclectic—and truly he well deserves that title, if truth is to be sacrificed to authority, and antiquity is to take precedence of observation. He borrowed from Bellini, the doctrine of obstruction, and with that error mingled from the same most astute genius, the fallacy of lentor, which Bellini had taken from the Cartesians. From Sylvius de le Boe, the archchemical pathologist, Boerhave derived the ridiculous figment of acid and alkali in the blood; and from the Galenical theory, he took the doctrine of plethora— and thus the mechanicians, cartesians and chemists, not furnishing to this eclectic error and folly, enough from which to fabricate a composite structure of idle and illusive explication of the nature of disease, the venerable Galen must be called on for aid, to help out the scheme. We fancy that we hear the grave and most renowned Boerhave soliloquizing, and thus addressing the manes of Bellini, de Boe and Galen, in the words of Prince Hal to Hotspur:

> " All the budding honours on thy crest
> I 'll crop, to make a garland for my head.

But that garland has withered, and so may all such false medical doctrines perish, amid the light and glory of advancing science!

The theory of his medicatrix naturæ, as enforced and relied upon by some authorities, partakes much of the mystical jargon of Stahl's Anima Medica. Dr. Cullen had the penetration to perceive this, and the candour to acknowledge it. "I might," says that great man, " go further, and show how much the atten-

5

tion to the autocrateia, allowed of in one shape or other, by every sect, has corrupted the practice among all physicians, from Hippocrates to Stahl. It must, however, be sufficiently obvious; and I shall conclude the subject with observing, that although the vis medicatrix naturæ must, unavoidably, be received as a fact; yet, wherever it is admitted, it throws an obscurity upon our system; and it is only where the impotence of our art is very manifest and considerable, that we ought to admit of it in practice."*

There are three very important admissions in the above passage, which should forever banish the doctrine of the vis medicatrix naturæ, or autocrateia, from medical philosophy. First, this doctrine has corrupted the practice of medicine among all physicians. Secondly, it throws an obscurity upon the system of medical science: And, thirdly, it should not be received, except in cases of such utter imbecility in our resources to conduct the treatment of disease, as to demand the interference of such a deity. But Horace's rule, nec deus intersit, nisi dignus, &c., would apply here with great force, and lead us to exclude all such vain and shadowy speculations.

The doctrine of the corruption of the blood in diseased states of the economy is amenable to one unanswerable objection—this corruption has never been demonstrated. It is surely not logical to contend for the possibility of a thing which has never been proven. We are not, as medical philosophers, to establish any

* Thompson's edition of Cullen's Works—Introductory Lecture—vol. 1st, p. 406.

of our views of morbid action on mere possible contin-
gencies. Cullen confesses that "these possible changes
of the fluids is seldom understood, and more seldom is
it known when they have taken place; that our reason-
ings concerning them have been, for the most part,
purely hypothetical, *have contributed therefore nothing to improve,* and have often misled the practice
of physic."

The above concession of this erudite teacher of medicine bears Sir Gilbert Blane out in the declaration that,
" the whole of the humoral pathology rested on a fallacious and shallow, though specious foundation."

A boundless terra incognita, as I have stated in
another place,* is presented by the mass of circulating
vital fluid, contained in the arteries and veins of the
animal machine, which our fond visionaries and
romance writers on medicine have peopled with every
variety of direful foes, to the weal of the body. Sometimes animalcula are made to sport in cruel triumph
along the conduits of life; at other times, the blood
is wrought into woful chemical changes, and is thick-
ened into a dark spissitude or lentor, or thinned into a
mere cruor, according as the mind of the medical
novelist is troubled with "thick coming fancies," or
is elated by etherial visions. One will gravely write
by the hour, of impregnations, foreign infusions, and
certain mysterious, but yet unappreciable changes in
the vital fluid. Another will dwell with infinite com-
placency on the horrible blackness of the blood, which

* Harrison on Cholera—Baltimore Medical and Surgical Journal; July 1834.

he finds dark as Cerberus, and fit only for congestions, collapses and death.   But a still additional writer shall entertain his readers, very little at his own expense of research, by expatiating over the ground of an ill-defined and misty space, from which he imagines he descries in clear perspective, both territories of humoralism and solidism.   Such a ready scribe speaks you fair, and tells you in grandiloquent phrase, of the possibilities, nay, absolute probabilities, of the blood becoming corrupted, and refers you for proof, not to the chemical analysis of any poisonous products found in the circulating mass, but to the experiments of some gentle vivisectors, who veritably force, by their torturing process, foreign materials into the blood vessels.   Medicine is *called* by these gentlemen, a demonstrative science—aye, they emblazon it by the proud titles of an inductive and certain science,— a department of human knowledge, requiring at each step of its glorious march to ultimate perfection, a precision in the collocation of its facts, and a fixedness in its positions, that can never be impaired by the revolutions of time.   Fond conceit ! 'Is not instability written on the face of our science, and shall they who yet foster the prejudices of the past, in favour of a doctrine that never has been proved, idly dream of the ultimate achievements of truth over error, when they are engaged in rebuilding the crumbling fabric reared in the dark ages of human knowledge!   We demand the proofs—we require, before we give our belief to the undigested doctrines of humoralism, to see something like a rigid and scientific appeal made to analysis and demonstration.   Who ever appeals to the chemical changes of the elementary constituents of the blood, either during life, or after death, for evidences of the state of morbid action that may be present, or has left its ravages behind? It is evident that an incalculable amount of false experience in medicine, must have been reared upon the conceptions of disease, and the modus agendi of remedial agents, adopted by the defenders of the humoral doctrine;—such conceptions, in the language of Cullen, having contributed nothing to improve, and having often misled the practice of physic.

Andral, who, to a very limited extent, is a humoralist, candidly avers, " that in the present state of the science, it is the part of a sensible man not to adopt the doctrine of humorism too lightly, by judging from facts, many of which require a re-examination before they are finally admitted, and that we ought to be particularly on our guard against being in too great a hurry to make practical applications of it."*

A doctrine so mysterious and impracticable, which must be thus guarded, limited and dreaded, lest we rashly employ it for any useful practical purpose, cannot, surely, derive its existence from correct and enlightened experience; and therefore, if we desire to see the reign of a just philosophy extending its healthful protection over the science of medicine, we should renounce a scheme of explanation of disease, which is not founded on sound observation, and which exerts such dubious, if not dangerous, tendencies over the practice of our art.

Methods of acquiring true experience.—There are two main sources opened to us for the attainment of

---

* Andral's Anatomy, vol. I. p. 419.

true experience in medicine. The one direct, emanating from our own personal observation; the other deriva-tive, flowing from the testimony of others. It requires but little reflection to convince the most obtuse mind that the last is the most copious and opulent source; that standing on that elevation we see centuries placed be-neath the eye, little names are obscured, things are ad-justed to a true point of comparison, and the glaring colours of present fashionable doctrines are effaced. To this point nothing should ascend but the spirit and true quality of medical truths. The science of medicine may be divided into principles and practice. Although for the purpose of a more easy and perspicuous discussion, such a division may be adopted, yet as a useful and ne-cessary art which is constantly operating on the dearest earthly interests of society, such an arbitrary separation between the principles and practice should not obtain. True experience is founded on a close union of the two; for without principles medicine is but a mechanical trade, and without practice those principles degenerate into idle speculations. What is so frequently called ex-perience, deserves not that appellation. *The wise only profit by experience,* is an adage that receives its most emphatic illustration in medicine. A man ignorant of the fundamental principles of the science, and incapable of reasoning in a correct manner, may grow gray in the practice, and remain ignorant of the most important truths. How often the hoary head of inveterate error occupies the chair of authority, which wisdom alone should fill. The most profoundly ignorant of medicine are often those who have paced along the deep worn path of routine for near half a century. A thorough indoctrination of the principles of medicine; an extensive, accurate, and profound medical erudition, are absolutely demanded to qualify men to acquire knowledge from their own observations. In vain are facts presented to the eye of one ignorant of the principles of our science; he is not capable of perceiving their import nor of deducing from them those corollaries which will guide him in future cases. There are no two cases of disease which bear an exact veri-similitude to each other in every respect. The endless varieties observed in different patients suffering under the same malady, arise from difference of constitution, diversity in modes of life, from the distinct nature of the exciting cause, and from the peculiar emotions which may at the time agitate the mind. To prescribe, therefore, the same remedies for the same disease without a due inquiry into the state of the system, merely because they were successful in another patient, is rank empiricism. A perception of analogy and contrariety must guide the practitioner in all new cases. Possessed of an accurate knowledge of the structure and functions of the healthy human body, and having acquired from his derivative experience a just conception of the nature, symptoms and treatment of the species of disease, to which the case under his observation belongs, the physician is well prepared to administer, not for the name of the malady, but for the state of the system.

There are three modes in which the mind acts in its acquisition of true experience, from personal observation. By the spirit of observation it collects the elements of judgment; by the force of its judgment it incorporates those elements, and by its creative energy it models and realizes new and felicitous combinations of thought. The spirit of observation is the messenger of reason, sent out before to explore and prepare the way: by it we penetrate into the phenomena of nature, and by the judgment and creative power of the mind we appropriate all that is gathered by observation, to the formation of a calm and contemplative turn of thought, which is not easily misled by the glare of novelty, nor seduced by the erring lights of a false experience.

By what preparatory steps, then, shall the mind be best qualified to profit by clinical observation? In answer to this question I reply, that it is, 1st. By a careful sedulity of effort in obtaining correct views of the anatomy and physiology of the human system. 2d. By ascertaining from books and lectures an accurate knowledge of remedies. 3d. By deriving experience from the testimony of judicious writers and lecturers on medicine.

The science of medicine, being the result of the accumulated knowledge of many cultivated reflecting minds, must be digested and arranged in accordance with a just order and perspicuous method, that it may become attainable by those, who may addict themselves to its study. It has, as a physical science, nothing directly to do with the knowledge of reasons and their conclusions, which constitutes abstract science; but is exclusively conversant with the investigation of causes, and their effects, and of the laws of nature. Whatever may be the value of the abstract sciences, the objects of which are those primary existences and relations, such as space, time, number, and order, and those artificial symbols, which the intellect creates, as representatives of its own conceptions, in disciplining thought, in developing the capacities of reason, and in imparting accuracy and precision to the communication of our ideas, still medicine owes little or nothing to the direct lights of the abstract sciences.

The foundation of all correct medical and surgical knowledge is anatomy. Disease is the product of disordered action in the living moving powers of the body. Disordered action cannot be understood without a knowledge of healthy function; healthy function cannot be understood without a correct knowledge of structure; and structure cannot be understood without investigating the anatomy of the system. The disordered movements of function can only be controlled by touching the springs of life. From the composite mechanism of the human body, and from the concealment of that mechanism from common observation, it requires an assiduous examination of the interior structure of each organ, vessel, nerve and tissue, in order to understand the relative situation and connexion, the nature and operation of the various parts of the frame liable to disease. In the pervading agency of the circulation, and the dominant influence exerted by the nervous system on all the actions of life, we see the immeasurable importance of a correct knowledge of these two great systems, in order understandingly to administer to cases in which they are involved in disease. And what disease is there in which they are not involved? Let one illustration suffice. When the liver is diseased there is often pain at the top of the shoulder. How is this to be accounted for by a man ignorant of anatomy? Such a man knows nothing of the right phrenic nerve which sends a branch to the liver, nor of the third cervical nerve, from which the phrenic arises, distributing branches to the neighbourhood of the shoulder; thus establishing a nervous communication between the shoulder and liver. Disease of the liver is sometimes treated by ignorant physicians as rheumatism of the shoulder.

To the surgeon, anatomy is all in all. It is what Bacon called knowledge in general; it is power in every sense of the word—power to prevent, power to alleviate, and power to save. Without anatomical knowledge, the surgeon is like a mariner on the sea without compass, chart, or the stars of heaven to guide him in a stormy night. The great improvements in surgery have invariably proceeded from the best informed anatomists. Surgery has risen to the certainty and perfection of its present condition by the cultivation of anatomy. John Hunter, the light and glory of English surgery, was the greatest anatomist of his age. Philip Syng Physick, the light and glory of American surgery, received his elementary knowledge in anatomy from Hunter.

The diffusive lustre of French Pathological and minute Anatomy, has shed the rays of a better philosophy on clinical experience. Commencing with the powerful and penetrating genius of Bichat, it has gone on to a more exalted position of usefulness. The physician who is ignorant of the researches of Bichat, and of the other authors who have written on minute and pathological anatomy, is ill prepared for profiting by his own observation. Such a one is destitute of the true elements of a correct clinical experience. He is like a man who attempts to construct an edifice without a knowledge of the rules of architecture; or like one who essays to solve an algebraical problem when he has omitted one of the elements of the calculation.

It is absolutely required as a preparation of mind for the obtainment of a sober experience of the remedial power of the different articles of the materia medica, that the physician should be versant in the history of the science. History is philosophy teaching by example. When we read of the numberless articles which have been obtruded on the medical world as rare and effective remedies in many diseases—when we read of the undistinguishing eulogies passed on inert medicines, and learn the adventitious fallacy connected with the reputed experience which gave them birth, we are made wise by such examples, and acquire that philosophical wariness of mind which leads us to listen with some considerable degree of scepticism to the accounts given of any new and extraordinary medicine. The history of the materia medica is little else than a history of false experience. The stream of time has washed away the dissoluble reputation of the great majority of articles once held in high estimation. A few are seen standing erect in the flood, and upon them is affixed the sure seal of an approved experience.

Amidst the wide spread triumphs of the art of printing, it were a superfluous task to attempt any commendation of the inestimable value of that transmitted experience, which we find recorded in books. Medicine is as deeply indebted to the art of printing for its present elevation and usefulness as any other tentative and progressive branch of knowledge. Cicero said, that the man who knew nothing of the past by reading, was always a child. And so it is in medicine; the physician who is uninstructed in the history of his science, and who expatiates on his own narrow field of observation, without deriving any light from his predecessors, or cotemporaries in medicine, is likely to remain a child in true experience all his days. To be sure he may have all the confidence which a true experience should alone give, yet it is the blind assurance of ignorant arrogance, not the firm dignity of conscious acquirement.

True experience does not always grow with the progress of years. In many instances advancing years but confirm the decisions of prejudice, and add strength to the presumptuousness of ignorance. Neither does the multitude of patients which a physician may be called to attend, necessarily enlarge his views, or add to the vigour of his judgment. It is not the number of cases which a physician sees, but the degree of careful analysis which he makes of those which are submitted to his inspection, which constitutes true experience. What is it that distinguishes the observing traveller from the undiscerning one? They both visit the same spots, and yet one will only tell you of things which interest you not, whilst the other, by leading you through the region of life and manners, will invigorate your intellect, and send a refreshing influence through every recess of thought. And what is it that made a Newton see an apple fall with a different eye from the millions who had witnessed the same phenomenon before? It was the power of perception, which dwelt in his inquisitive

and penetrating mind, that separated him so far from
the generality of mankind. And what is it that distinguishes the physician from the nurse, but the disparity
existing in the degree of their mental cultivation ? The
nurse is in possession of the same senses by which the
phenomena of disease are discerned as the physician;
and yet the pure emanations of an enlightened reason
and a true experience, are the product of the observations, and of the theoretic views of the one, whilst the
gross and vulgar apprehensions of the other seem more
like the limited, instinctive perceptions of the lower
animals.

To the formation of a sound discriminating judgment
in practical medicine, there can be no substitute for
clinical observation. Whatever attainments the student may make in anatomical, physiological, and pathological knowledge, still he must have his faculties exercised at the bedside, to enable him to acquire a just and
useful experience in the art of curing disease. There
can be no substitute for this most essential mode of
gaining a knowledge of the symptoms and nature of
the various maladies to which the human economy is
subject. All other acquisitions are only preparatory
to the acquirement of clinical experience. Without
witnessing the diversified phases of disease, as they
reveal themselves substantially and truly at the suffering patient's couch, all our attainments, however valuable as a preparation, are useless as an end. As a terminating point of practical utility, it is very patent to the
most obtuse intellect, that the most accurate views of
the organization of man's composite frame, or of the
laws of healthy action established in that organization,

or even of the laws of morbid action, could never impart enlightened views of the symptomatology and therapeutics of disease. No one can be a scientific physician unless he is intimately acquainted with the anatomy and physiology of the body—but neither can he be a judicious and safe practitioner, unless he super-adds to all such most necessary preparatory knowledge, the knowledge of disease as it is derivable from seeing it—and of realizing its presence and power, and many changes, by an actual examination of the suffering fellow being, whose system is prostrate under its powerful agency. We can not insist too strenuously on this point—it is of vital consequence to the growth of a legitimate experience in medicine,—and without it, without clinical observation—whatever embellishments collateral branches of knowledge may pour around our art—whatever most necessary investigations may be had into anatomy, physiology and pathology, as these fundamental divisions of our science are learned in dissection, lectures and books, yet at last the student of medicine must acquire for himself, by an exploration of the phenomena of disease at the bedside, the crowning excellence of all useful experience. Anatomy must be known, not merely by a careful perusal of authors, or by attendance on demonstrations of the anatomical theatre, but by dissection. Books and lectures are well—are needful—but dissection is better, and more needful. Physiology is more dependent on books for its inculcation—but let the student not linger too long in the enchanting bowers of physiological speculation. How much is written on physiological topics,—and written with great plausibility and eloquence too—that is the mere bodying forth of a vivid imagination. Pathology must be studied in books, lectures, and by post mortem examinations. It is apparent that as anatomy is dependent on a special method of inquiry—that by dissection for its cultivation—and as physiology and pathology, are each to be learned in accordance with their peculiar modes of investigation—so must a just knowledge of disease be attained. We must see disease before we practically can know what are its phenomena, the fluctuations incident to it, and the effects wrought upon it by our remedies. To approach the bedside with every advantage for a skilful exploration of the symptoms, the student is to be well grounded in the precognita of the science—these precognita are, as already stated—anatomy, physiology and pathology. Anatomy, both special and general, as well as pathological, must be well comprehended before the inquirer at the bedside can stand on sure ground in his interpretation of morbid phenomena. And anterior to a fair construction of the intensity of the deviations from healthy action observed in the system labouring under disordered and irregular movements, the observer must know what constitutes physiological appearances. But there may be an excessive refinement in anatomical researches, at war with the results flowing from the general and pervading harmony of the parts constituting the organism. Thus let us take the brain and its investments for an illustration. The substance of the brain, as an integral mass, may be looked at in three aspects. First, the brain; and in this consideration 1 include the spiral marrow, may be regarded as the controlling organ of all nervous influence. Se-

condly, we may consider the encephalon as the instrument of mental operations. And thirdly, we may
simply view the brain as the fountain-head of nervous
influence to animal life, or to the organs of relation.
Now it is very clear that either of these views of the
brain may be pronounced just, if not too isolated. Sup-
pose we contemplate the brain in the first light, as the
controlling organ of all nervous influence: this view
must be met and modified by the third aspect, in which
the importance of the organ is to be recognized. For
although man cannot live without the influence of the
brain, yet the ganglionic system subserves such an important purpose in our economy, as to evince that a
low degree of life can be sustained even in man, when
the functions of the brain are greatly abridged. Some
physiologists, more addicted to intangible speculations
than beseems an inquiry so dependent on proof for
substantiation as the question under consideration, have
regarded the brain, to use an expression of Broussais,
as an "ontological republic," divided off into so many
compartments; and to each compartment, they appropriate the residence of a particular faculty of the mind.
We object to this scheme of explanation of diseases of
the mind, not because it does not explain some of the
difficulties in the way of a correct conception of insanity in its varied shades, but because it pretends to
cover a field which it does not half occupy; and because
it leaves out of its most gratuitous hypothesis any philosophical reference to the effects of distant organs on
the encephalon. Mental aberration is often induced by
irritation of the stomach, or uterus, or any important
viscus, or by a general derangement of the system. If

the view controverted, be true, how does one compartment of the brain receive the irritation from the suffering organ, and not the other compartments? There is
no particular nerve given off from such a portion of the
general mass of the cerebral substance, that could be
the special conveyancer of that irritation? Besides, in
conducting the treatment of insanity, no such wire-
drawn reflections can conduce to our safe guidance
along the path of a judicious practice. And so with
regard to the other aspects, presented briefly above, in
which the brain is to be considered. Too abstract a
conception of the functions of the encephalon, must not
be taken in the treatment of disease—they are important in anatomy and physiology, to simplify the materials of study, and to render the perquisition of these
branches of knowledge more accessible, but if too
rigidly carried out into our practical conceptions of
morbid action, they will mislead.

The brain and its membranes are not to be too sys-
tematically and rigidly separated in our investigations
of disease. Serres has attempted this with regard to
apoplexy, and has erected a division of that affection,
upon a supposed disparity of the phenomena generated
by inflammation of the membranes, contradistinguished
from structural lesion of the substance of the brain.
But his division is not generally regarded as founded
upon just experience. The immense advantages that
have accrued to practical medicine from minute pathological anatomy should not render us insensible to the
errors which may spring from a too exclusive study of
disease through that channel of inquiry. Symptomatology must be studied most carefully, but always in

connexion with pathological anatomy, and, whilst the
student of medicine assiduously strives to accumulate
the stores of a scientific knowledge of his profession,
let him ever keep in mind that at the bed side, in actual
contact with disease, in the wards of a hospital, or the
private chambers of the sick, must be gathered the elements of a legitimate experience.   The effects of remedies can be learned only by fair and repeated trials of
their virtues in disease.   No analysis of their constituent principles can ever assure us of their modes of action in the eradication of a deranged condition of the
vital actions.   Neither can their potency, or impotency
in disease be known by experiments upon the human
body in health.   Nor can the agency of a remedy in
any given malady be confidently predicted by our past
experience of that remedy in another dissimilar affection.   We should not allow any a priori views to
darken our observations at the bed side. We must come
to the study of disease, its symptoms, and the effects of
remedial measures on its progress, with minds unbiased
by any preconceptions of the modus agendi of the
means to be employed.   Incalculable mischief is done
by a violation, reckless and obstinate, of this obvious
suggestion of true experience.   Thus in Paris, the
bright and glorious city of intellectual scepticism and
pride, the astounding anomaly, during the prevalence
of cholera there, was witnessed, of a total exclusion of
calomel from the treatment of that fatal epidemic.
Leeches, tea, lemonade, enemata, punch, iced water,
and weak coffee—these were relied on by such men as
Lisfranc, Bouilland, Piorry and Broussais, to arrest
this most fatal malady; but calomel—that was not

even to be tried;—and why? because these gentlemen
had before trial, and in direct contradiction to the published experience of such men as Johnson, Orton,
Craigie and others, determined that calomel was too
irritating, or perturbating for cholera. We fear that
popular prejudice swayed their judgments more than
any reasoning on the subject; for the French seem to
regard calomel in the light of a pernicious drug, only
to be used to cure a still viler disease.

In the examination of disordered states of the animal
economy, three distinct and prominent points are to be
preserved in all our computations of the degree of danger involved in the case. First, Is the disease we are
surveying one of functional derangement, unaccompanied by structural alteration? Second, Has structural
lesion supervened on disordered function? And, third,
Has the functional ensued upon the structural disease?
The neuralgic affections, and some cases of fever, are
instances of simply disordered function. Tetanus and
hydrophobia are so likewise, for no satisfactory local
alteration of structure has been identified as standing in
the relation of invariable antecedent to either disease,
in a pathological point. In many, not all, cases of idio-
pathic fever, we find, after death, structural disease following constitutional functional derangement. Severe
constitutional irritation will, upon reaction, induce local
changes of the interior organs. Burns, especially in
children, will frequently produce, just on the eve of
their cure, inflammation of the pleura, or arachnoid
membrane.

The phlegmasiæ, as well as accidents inflicting injury
on the extremities, are followed by functional disease.

Pleurisy, or pneumonia, furnish an illustration relevant to the above remark. When therefore we come to the bed side we must conduct our examination of the case with special reference to the above considerations. Is the patient affected with local disease—and is that a functional one? Or has he a functional malady terminating in alteration of some organ? Or has the affection been originally a structural one, and does it now implicate the most important functions? What is the state of the head—of the organs of the chest—of those of the abdomen—in what condition is the skin—what is the degree of oppression and debility under which he labours, and how do the remedies administered operate? These general questions must be met, and satisfactorily answered in the mind of the practitioner, before he prescribes. Nor must the decubitus, and physiognomy of the patient be overlooked. The station occupied by the medical adviser at the side of the suffering fellow being is full of solemn responsibility. He is called upon by the august voice of humanity, and by the stern monitions of an enlightened conscientiousness, to spare no pains in the scrutiny exercised by his mind upon the state of his patient. Then having satisfied his judgment as to the condition and danger of the case, let his mind be pregnant with expedients for the mitigation of pain, the extinction of disease, and the prolongation of life, thus proving that our art is the handmaid of nature, in a wise interpretation of her laws, and a sedulous guidance of the actions of life to a restoration from an irregular discharge of its functions to accustomed health.

From what has been said it appears that true experience is to be acquired by a careful avoidance of those sources of error, fallacy, and misapprehension, whence false experience springs, by a well grounded knowledge of the elementary branches of medical science, and by the exercise of a discriminating observation upon the phenomena submitted to personal inspection.

But if the physician permits his mind to be preoccupied with any shadowy and airy notions of congestion, or any other universal all-embracing, all-explaining, and at the same time vague and indefinite, a priori views, of disease, in vain opportunities, the most ample and diversified, of acquiring a correct experience are presented.

Such a one sees his predominant image of mind reflected in every symptom—all phases of disease are but the variegated aspects of the ruling figment of his mind, and like a man with a calenture on the brain, he peoples vacuity itself with the creation of his prolific fancy: or with Wirdig he runs into the extravagance of endeavouring to explain every thing in heaven and earth, and under the earth, by his favourite hypothesis. Thus that erring philosopher asserted of magnetism, "Universa natura magnetica est; totus mundus constat et positus est in magnetismo, omnes sublunariæ vicissitudines fiunt per magnetismum; vita conservatur magnetismo, interitus omnium rerum fiunt per magnetismum."

Such a habit of mind converts knowledge into prejudice, and limits every intellectual exercise within the narrow boundaries of a crude and indigested hypothesis. Our ideas should be daily subjected to new developments, and knowledge acquired by past observations must be constantly quickened and made prolific of new trains of thought by incessant efforts of improvement. Let us beware of a desire to subsist all our lives on the acquisitions of a few years study and experience; let us not exist in a state of mental petrifaction—preserving a lifeless form of medical experience, without the animating spirit of discovery, but uniting the acquisitions gathered from the past with the accessions of each revolving day, we shall rise higher and higher in the scale of improvement, and become more firmly fixed on the ground of true medical experience.

Should the student of medicine feel as deep an interest in the subject discussed, in the foregoing pages, as its inherent merit demands, he will seek a more enlarged acquaintance with it. That such a mental want on his part may be met, and receive its adequate supply, I will refer him to the best sources for information on this thesis. The learned Zimmerman has written two volumes on Medical Experience, replete with much that is instructive on various medical topics, but deficient in direct and obvious bearing on the particular theme of his inquiry. The judicious Cullen has many just thoughts, in the introductory part of his Materia Medica, on the intellectual wariness and wise scepticism, which we should ever exercise in reference to the reputed efficacy of remedies. Paris has, in part, followed Zimmerman in the order of his reflections on the causes which have impeded the march of curative medicine; but the train of thought pursued by him is far superior in practical good sense, and enlightened discrimination to that so tediously indulged in by his predecessor. Sir Gilbert Blane, in his Medical Logic, has communicated many suggestions on the subject of medical experience, which are pregnant with the soundest philosophy. Some of his illustrations are inapposite, and badly selected; but his small work is one of great merit, being opulent in the copious contributions of a gifted and cultivated mind. Dr. Abercrombie, in his work on the Intellectual Powers, has given some excellent rules by which the medical student should be guided in his investigations. There are very few writers in our profession, who possess faculties better disciplined for the discovery of truth than this distinguished author. All that he has written bears the clear impress of a sound and vigorous intellect, cultivated to a skilful action of its powers on the rich field of medical knowledge. In an eminent degree he stands equally in contrast with an addictedness to impracticable speculations on the one hand, and to a blind fondness for the application of general rules and deductions on the other. His distinguishing qualities are patience of labour, sagacity of observation, sound judgment, and practical tact, with a pervading spirit of common sense discipline of mind, binding in harmony, and inspiriting with life, his other powers.

ADDRESS,

DELIVERED BEFORE THE LOUISVILLE MEDICAL
SOCIETY, AT THEIR ANNUAL MEETING,
JANUARY 1, 1833.

Gentlemen of the Louisville Medical Society:

The economy of human life seems to consist of wants,
with their correlative supplies, and of evils with their
corresponding remedies. The evil of sickness is in-
separable from our mortal condition, and it becomes a
want of pressing urgency to seek, in the art of healing,
for methods of relief. Among a rude and uncivilized
people, this art is limited to a few crude and simple prescriptions, but in proportion to the progress of social
refinement, medicine assumes the dignity of a distinguished science, difficult of attainment, and characterized by the diversified application of its means for the
cure of disease. Medicine is a science of well ascertained and carefully collected facts. It is indebted for
its present elevation among the other branches of human knowledge to the Baconian method of discovering
truth, so successfully pursued in all physical investigations. The art of restoring health, took its rise in
necessity; the first methods adopted for relief in pain
were, perhaps, prompted by instinct; these were im-

proved upon as chance suggested the efficacy of other remedies, after repeated trials of which, observation either confirmed, or annulled, the propriety of their further employment. Analogy aided in the more extensive application of the remedial plans, adopted with success in simple and common departures from health, to morbid affections of rare occurrence, and of more difficult treatment. By analogy, likewise, plants, possessing taste, smell and appearance similar to those already in use as medicines, were brought into requisition, and their virtues tested by experiment. Experience, which means nothing more than repeated observation on the curative measures instituted for the restoration of health, is assuredly at the foundation of all successful practice in medicine. But then it is an experience not limited to a physician's own circumscribed sphere of observation; but an experience enlarged and liberalized by study, by reflection, and careful comparison. There should be no controversy on this point among well-informed physicians. True experience consists in accurate and correct observation. A previous cultivation of mind on the fundamental branches of medical science; a thorough and well grounded knowledge of the structure of man; a comprehensive acquaintance with the laws which govern life, with the modes in which modifications of vital action ensue from the impressions, within and without the system, constantly made on these laws, are indispensable præcognita to the acquisition of a true, sound and valuable experience. But the mental process, the induction and analysis, carried on by two different medical practitioners of equal opportunities of experience, may differ as much

7

as wisdom differs from folly. Here is the point upon which, at last, rests all the acquirements of a true experience in medicine. For if there be no sagacity, no power of penetrating inspection, and of correct inference, in the mind of the physician, of what avail is it that he has trod a wide field of practice, in which he has stumbled over the most ample and varied opportunities of improvement? But to a man gifted with an original capacity of inquiry, sharpened in its discernment by a liberal culture of the faculties, of great vigilance in the exercise of observation, and of a strong, and strenuously exerted power of generalization on the facts before him, a very short time may be sufficient to supply a large share of the knowledge, derivable from experience. Such a physician will be rich in the benefits of sound experience, and possess the judgment and decision legitimately founded on that accomplishment long before he has attained old age. Thus exemplifying the wise and beautiful remark, that wisdom is gray hair to man, and an unspotted life is old age.

Medicine is neither a finished, nor a perfect science. It is not finished, because it still admits of an increase of light, certainty and power. It is not perfect, otherwise, no doubts would be entertained on the nature and treatment of any disease, which physicians are called upon to cure. And because it is neither a finished, nor a perfect science, we are assembled together this evening as a voluntary association, formed for our mutual improvement in medical knowledge. The world is always better for every provocative to good thoughts and designs, by which its intelligence may be augmented and its aims exalted. And the science of medi-

cine is quickened in its career of advancement by a
friendly interchange of facts, and an intercommunion of
thought, on medical subjects, between cultivated physicians. By the shock of fair and enlightened discussion
truth is elicited; facts seen by one are made known to
other minds, and a deeper interest is created in the observation and generalization of the phenomena presented
at the bed side of the sick. As members of a medical
society, we wish to test our opinions and modes of
practice by the views entertained by each other, and to
receive such accession of facts and views on the topics
brought up for discussion as to enlarge the boundaries
of our theoretic knowledge, and impart greater certainty to our plans of treating diseases. We believe
that we are neither too wise, nor too old to learn. We
believe that our science needs many contributions from
its members in order to give more comprehension and
precision to its institutes, and to reduce to order and
system, the contradictory plans employed to restore the
disordered actions of the body. Experience we re-
cognize as valuable, but in our discussion on points of
practice, there is not a member of our society who
would have intellectual boldness enough to set aside the
experience of the profession at large, or erect his own
comparatively slender experience in opposition to that
of the most distinguished men in the profession, both at
home and abroad, who, either are now alive, or have
belonged to past times. Nor does our desire for additional light, and our deference for authority, spring
from an entire renunciation of our own opinions. We
are deeply impressed with the importance of as complete an acquaintance with every medical subject as our

opportunities of observation, our perusal of authors, and an interchange of opinion between each other, will admit, to enable our minds to form the best judgment at which we can arrive. A man conscious of the independence of his views, who can rely on the operations of his own faculties, is not afraid to receive the opinions of others. He listens with attention to what may be advanced, and uses it as counsel, but does not submit to it as so authoritative as to suspend the exercise of his judgment, or supersede his reasoning powers. But he whose views stand in jeopardy every hour of being confounded by objections, and who avoids the collision of other minds, because his opinions are liable to be driven about by every breath of opposition, had better never attach himself to any society in which free, fair, and fearless controversy is conducted. Such a society affords an excellent arena on which the soundness of medical doctrines is tested. It opens a field for the exhibition of extensive professional acquirements. Within its consecrated enclosure there is breathed upon each member a kindling influence to prompt to higher acquisitions of medical knowledge. Each one belonging to such a society, who feels the impulses of a laudable ambition, and who is embued with the true spirit of the association, has strong desires animating his mind not to appear ignorant in such a circle. For he is aware that the judgment passed by medical men on the attainments of a physician is the only true standard of his merit. The motives, thus derived, do not cease in their exciting influence, with the discussions of the evening. They abide in living constancy, instinct with urgent aspirings after additional light, during the days which intervene between the meeting. They urge to industry and diligence in the study of our science, impart fresh interest to the most common cases of sickness which we are called to treat, and spread a softening charm over all the difficulties experienced in our professional course. By such a society the esprit du corps is kept alive among its members; by which zeal for the common honour, they are preserved from a misunderstanding of each other's character, and from those jealousies which are such a fruitful source of professional enmities. We have need of every auxiliary motive, not drawn directly from a sense of our responsibility, to sustain our unfaltering way amidst the many and severe discouragements which impede our professional career.

Every profession is what its members choose to make it. If the medical profession is filled with ignorant, conceited, and immoral men, it must soon become degraded in the eyes of society. Thus degraded, the community must reap the bitter fruits which grow on such a poisonous tree. There must be physicians—and the only question to be settled by men of virtue and intelligence is, whether it is best to have an ignorant, crafty and dishonest set of medical advisers, or men of cultivation, of integrity, and of liberal deportment, to administer to them when ill. It would seem that this question is of easy solution; but the patronage afforded vile empiricism by men who pass for enlightened, throws ominous perplexity on the matter. Ignorance is universally conceded to be pernicious to the welfare of society. And yet with this general admission, ignorance is every day encouraged by the most extravagant praise. Not as ignorance, it is true, but cloaked in the bold, assumptions of superior skill, is it patronized in preference to knowledge, unaccompanied by that self-commendation and self-glorification, which are the current language of quackery. The atmosphere around us appears congenial to vapours and false fires. The lights of our profession shed a feeble ray on eyes blinded by the glare of such false fires. But let us not yield to the disheartening considerations thus derived. Let us be encouraged by every motive drawn from the cause of humanity, from a sense of responsibility, and from the unbought pleasures of a conscientious feeling of manly adherence to the best of causes. Pursued in the legitimate spirit of its high and liberal tendency, medicine is a science of great dignity and importance. It connects itself to the best interests of man; is conversant with the noblest piece of mechanism which God has framed; enters into the retirements of sickness, and often snatches the victim of disease from a premature grave. The enlightened physician is an humble imitator of Heaven, who sends his blessings on the evil and the good. Medicine is a liberal profession. The physician should be a man of letters. Liberal learning ought to be a constituent of his professional character. Medicine opens to the intellect, a wide range—a range commensurate with man in the most extended relations of his being. It is the testimony of a late most eloquent writer,* that the medical profession has furnished more examples of active and enlightened humanity than any other walk or profession. Aside from the direct ministrations of skill, the enlightened physician can aecom-

* Robert Hall.

plish much for the cause of science and humanity. The examples of such men as Boerhave, Sydenham, Rush and Wistar, illustrate and adorn the periods in which they lived, and send down the stream of time a pure and refreshing influence to quicken and rejoice future generations. Different departments of physical science are under great obligations to our profession for their cultivation. Chemistry, mineralogy, natural history and natural philosophy, have received many contributions from physicians. And medicine can enumerate a Goldsmith, an Aiken, an Aikenside, a Locke, a Brown and a Mackintosh, among the constellation of great men who have delighted and improved the world by their literary and metaphysical writings. It behoves us therefore to esteem our profession as one of dignity, of usefulness and of commanding importance in society. If it fall into dishonour and disrepute, the fault must lie on the heads of physicians. Let them watch assiduously over its character and reputation, maintain its standing by an honourable bearing and courageous consistency; preserve the parallelism of their course, undeterred by the froward petulance, and vain banter of the superficial, and scrupulously avoid every art of indirection and supplantation in order to acquire business. A resolute attachment to the higher functions of the profession is the best safeguard against that degrading rivalry in money making which inflicts such deep wounds on the medical character. An unalterable law of our moral nature—a law of continuity, or homogeneity, in the human mind—binds that physician down to a perpetual conscious self-degradation, who has spontaneously and deliberately violated those rules of professional ethics, which not only rest upon the rectitude and perspicacity of an enlightened judgment, but come recommended by the past and contemporary practice among the wisest and best members of our profession. The medical practitioner who connives at, or in ány manner encour- ages, quackery to day, will ever retain his own con- scious dereliction. He takes his permanent professional character from such a humiliation, to which he has submitted from considerations of the grossest self in- terest. On his own spirit he has brought a stain which time can never efface. His mind submissively bows to the humiliating terms by which he becomes a pensioner on the bounty of an abused CREDULITY—he sinks to the level of his lot, and even accepts and hails the scorn that belongs to it.

When practised in the genuine spirit of its character, medicine promotes every generous sentiment of human nature. It brings into play the finest feelings of sym- pathy, develops the noblest suggestions of a tender concern for human happiness, and fills the mind with an untiring ardour for the discovery and application of the most successful methods of alleviating pain, and re- moving disease.

The importance of our station in society should be felt and acknowledged in the beneficial effects flowing from our profession, rather than in any ostentatious mode of displaying it; and the consciousness of it, in- stead of evaporating in vain pretensions, should pro- duce a still more assiduous devotion of our time and concentration of our powers to its improvement. By an exalted appreciation of the science of medicine, we never can promote personal vanity among physicians.

From such a high estimate of our profession, we draw
incentives to a modest opinion of our present attainments. The standard of excellence being lifted up
above the ordinary rate of professional knowledge,
constantly reminds us of our deficiencies. Thus a pervading and influential persuasion of the contrast felt
between our acquisitions and the standard we have set
before us, leads the mind to that philosophical hu-
mility, which is at the foundation of all sound acquirements. The physician who does not possess this philosophical modesty, can entertain no correct conception
of abstract excellence in the line of his profession. He,
therefore, cannot hold converse with things greater
than those presented in the limited range of his own
ideas. His faculties never will stretch their energies in
an eager and untiring effort for additional illumination.
A meagre mind is apt to be filled with the turgid expansion of a spurious, affected greatness. A habit of
abstraction liberates the mental powers from that partial aspect and contracted estimate of the worth, and
dignity and utility of the healing art which so fix the
attention, enchain the faculties, and circumscribe the
exertions of many in our profession, that they seem to
regard the whole matter of medical science, in its
entire length and breadth, in its fulness of varied
research and minuteness of practical application, as of
very easy attainment. Where others toil with patient
force of investigation to acquire a knowledge of diseases with the best methods of curing them; their viva-
cions wits adopt a more compendious method. Such
practitioners look on an experience derived from prae-
tice as constituting the sum and substance of all medi-

cal knowledge. With them books are mere dull repo-
sitories of theoretic absurdities, and all discussion of
subjects connected with the science a waste of breath,
or a shock of adverse and irreconcilable dogmas. Reasoning in medicine they renounce and hold in utter
abhorrence, as being inconsistent with the unerring
decisions of their vigorous and untrammeled faculties.
From their fancied height of professional infallibility,
they look with pity, or contempt, on those who are
toiling in the barren region of doubt, or ascending the
rugged path of philosophical induction. Such men,
perhaps, have gathered up a few crude notions of disease from such books as Buchan's Medicine, and
Thomas's Practice, and these are fixed and perpetuated
in their minds, without the intrusion of other ideas.
The morning sun brings no new train of thought to
their torpid brains, and the evening rays depart, still
leaving them surrounded by the darkness of their
voluntary ignorance.

The science of medicine consists not solely in the
administration of a few remedies for some special cases
of disease, but in a wide and comprehensive acquaintance with the anatomy and physiology of man—of the
laws which govern the living organization—of the best
mode of preserving health, and of warding off attacks
of sickness, by a correct knowledge of the numerous
agents which are incessantly acting on the system.
The atmosphere, with its chemical constituents, and
its various impregnations of gaseous substances—the
quality and quantity of food—climate in its heat and
coldness, dryness and moisture—exercise and rest in
their invigorating and debilitating tendencies—sleep in

its refreshing and renovating power—the secretions and excretions, in their quality, quantity or absence—the reciprocal agency exerted by the mind and body on each other—and the dominant control often exercised by the moral emotions, either of a depressing or exciting kind—these and many other distinct topics of inquiry are continually presenting themselves to the mind of the physician, and demanding of him a careful and protracted research. These constitute but the alpha of the diversified points involved in the general consideration of the study of our science.

In seasons of epidemic visitations of some fatal malady, the transcendent importance of well-instructed and humane physicians is felt by society. The boastful quack, in such a time of panic and distress, like some bird of prey that hovers over a scene of destruction, is true to his end. He avails himself of the alarm and confusion of such a season, and spreads wide the meshes of his net to entrap the credulous and unwary. But the generous and enlightened physician gives up his mind to the most anxious thoughts, that he may arrest the destructive march of the pestilence; and if his plans of practice prove successful, he does not conceal them in mystery, but lays them before the public for their benefit.

The relation sustained by the physician towards his patient would seem to warrant the supposition that the perception of obligation on the part of the sick man would not soon fade from his mind. Other professional men advise, but the medical man prescribes. His authority over his patient is for the time, ascendant and complete. There is an implicitness of acquiescence on the suffering man's part which is not manifested in any other transaction of life. Yet how soon does the remembrance of services performed by the most skilful and humane physician, perish! With a waywardness, not displayed in other things, the medical man is often dismissed from his attendance on the sick, and all his assiduity is overlooked in the eager quest after some new physician, whose strongest claim upon public confidence, often consists in the confident averments made by himself of his superior ability in the cure of disease. In the "corrupted passages of this world," I am aware that it is scarcely possible for a man of the most cultivated intellect, and of the most honourable deportment to be much engaged in professional business without suffering from the injustice, caprice, and inconsideration of those with whom he is concerned. Calm reflection will teach him not to permit these evils, so incident to a responsible position in society, to agitate and disturb his tranquillity, or in any degree to turn him aside from a persevering prosecution of a useful scheme of life. A magnanimous spirit will not be subdued into a tame and servile compliance with wrong modes of gaining business by the success which accompanies the deceptious pretensions of those physicians, who abuse and delude the public by the arts and blandishments of quackery. Conscious rectitude, and an elevation of mind which despises such paltry shifts and devices, will sustain a man in the even tenor of his way far better than all the shouts of a misguided public.

We must allow human nature the liberty of some freaks and eccentricities in medical matters, as well as in religion and government. Men love the luxury of delusion, and possess a strong appetite for mystery. Let them be indulged to some extent, for they may more easily be exorcised of their delusion, after they are filled to satiety, with the diet with which imposture feeds the credulity of the simple. Various are the schemes by which empirical pretenders have endeavoured—too often with full success crowning their efforts—to raise a reputation, to attract employment, and to acquire an ascendency over their patients.* The

---

* "Whenever an individual," says an intelligent writer, in an excellent paper published in the North American Review, for July, 1828, "admits and acts upon the idea, that any other consideration than that of professional knowledge and worth is to be the chief measure or means of his success, he becomes accessible to motives which will almost inevitably lead into practices, dishonourable to himself and injurious to others. While that sound learning which, in its very nature, elevates the character, is neglected, those acts of winning popularity, which as certainly debase and disgrace it, are cultivated in its stead. He need not be an old man, who can remember when it was the general impression, throughout a great portion of our country, that the same course of preparatory education which was even then regarded as a necessary preliminary to entering upon the study of either of the other learned professions, was quite supererogatory in this. For our individual selves, though we lay no claim to the honours of ages, we have heard in our day a worthy member of a New England legislature speak with great contempt of the folly of sending a young man to attend a course of lectures, and declare that his son, who was to be a doctor, should go to a dancing master to learn the acts of ingratiating himself with his patients." "What more shameful," says a French writer, "what more dishonourable to science, and yet what more common, than to see men, who consider themselves in possession of good sense, reposing confidence

8

physician, who possesses true greatness of mind, whose
moral sensibility shrinks from the defilement contracted by meanness and disingenuousness, will never
degrade his profession by such acts as ignorant boldness employs to recommend itself to the patronage of
the public.   For he is assured, that after all, competent
ability, inflexible probity, diligence, humanity and
unaffected kindness, are the sure elements of his certain future elevation.   These qualities are the brightest
ornaments of the physician's character, and form the
best ground work upon which to build a lasting fame.
Even should a want of success now attend his strug-
gling steps, he will not abandon the firm foundation of
his hope of a final triumph over all the obstacles now
lying in his path.   He fears the check and rebukes of
a violated conscience more than poverty.   Relying on
the goodness of his cause, he feels assured that a final,
though long delayed, decision in favour of intelligence,
probity, and professional worth, will be made by the
public.   Filled with a rejoicing consciousness that

in mere pretenders to medicine, who are destitute of logic, and
ignorant sometimes of the first elements of grammar, under the
ridiculous pretext that such quacks may possess excellent receipts;
and that they have seen them effect wonderful cures!   The more
ignorant and presumptuous a man is, the more he inspires confidence in certain people.   A physician who has studied long to
acquire information has nothing marvellous about him; but the individual who can hardly speak his native tongue, has the reputation of knowing secrets which are omnipotent against most disorders; many see in him something wonderful, even supernatural; and
their confidence is strengthened by that which ought to destroy it."

when the hour of prosperity arrives he will be pre-
pareed to enjoy it with a purer and higher satisfaction
arising from his past course, he calmly awaits a turn in
the tide of events, which will sweep away the unwor-
thy adventurer in physic from his present moorings
into that ocean of hazardous enterprize for which his
spirit was framed.

Gentlemen, we are surrounded by a cloud of witnesses to our professional eminence. The bright constellation of illustrious men, who have died, covered
with the glory acquired in relieving the sufferings of
human nature, shed on our path their radiant example—
and invite us to a participation of their fame—society,
though at times unmindful of the obligations it is under
to our profession, expects of us a faithful performance
of the duties attached to the responsible stations we
occupy—the voice of humanity is borne by every sigh
that escapes the sick, and tells upon all the tender cha-
rities of our nature—the monitions of conscience impress us with a solemn feeling of our high calling, and
the more awful and awakening language which bursts
from the skies, resounds in our ears, inviting us by all
the rewards of a bright immortality, to fulfil the task
assigned us in mitigating wo, obeying the call of distress, rekindling the lamp of life ready to be extinguished by disease, and lighting up joy in a circle of
friends, whom the shade of death, approaching some
beloved object, had lately covered with sorrow. Then
will our success be signalized by the tears of gratitude,
the congratulations of friends, and the raptures of returning health, and with pure and unmingled satisfaction, we can taste of that divine felicity which springs
from the luxury of doing good.

REMARKS

ON THE INFLUENCE OF THE MIND UPON THE BODY:
AN INTRODUCTORY LECTURE, DELIVERED
MARCH 27, 1827.

To a Course of Clinical Lectures in the Louisville Hospital.

Fundamental to every process of reasoning, there are primary truths, which being admitted, without debate, become the ground work on which the whole superstructure is erected. Thus in an algebraical problem, certain elements are assumed; and in our discussions about the laws which regulate matter, we take it for granted, that matter does exist, and that it is known by certain properties. So in reference to the theme of inquiry now proposed, I regard the separate existence of the mind from the body, as a self-evident truth. For were I to contemplate the mind merely as a modified result of the organization of the body, there would be a palpable absurdity in attempting to show, that one portion of the body had an influence and agency upon another portion; there being a pervading influence of harmonious co-operation exerted upon the entire circle of the bodily organs.

But the mind, although in intimate union with the body, is yet a distinct entity. Though running in parallel lines with the body, and deeply implicated in all its movements, it still manifests a superior nature, and a far nobler destiny.

View man with a philosophic eye from the cradle to the grave! See him wailing his infant cries beneath the canopy of a mother's smiles, then behold the same being immured within the narrow confines of the sepulchre; and say, ye sage speculators! can you discover any thing, either at his birth, or in his meridian prime, or in his mournful exit from life, which furnishes you with convincing proof, that the mind is but a part of the frail body—that the jewel and the casket are the same!

It is the part of reason to draw deductions from premises made known, and infer sound conclusions from data indisputably established. But it is the part of madness, even to deduce sound conclusions from mistaken premises.

Reason should abstain from all presumptuous inference, where proof is not afforded. Now apply this rule of correct philosophizing to the subject of mind. We have no evidence that the mind and body are the same, and we should, therefore, not too confidently insist on a thing so uterly beyond our cognizance. Yet we have cogent proofs furnished, that the mind is governed by laws essentially distinct in nature from those which control our material fabric: that though a very intimate connection may exist between them, yet there is ample evidence to demonstrate that they are not identical. Connection will not prove identity; neither will the reciprocal agency of mind and matter on each other, establish, in the view of correct philoso-

phy, the opinion, that the mind is but a subtile, spirit-
ualized product of the brain.

A subject is known by its predicates. The body is
recognised by-its own properties; the mind is recognised by its own attributes. There is no sort of just
comparison between the properties of the one, and the
attributes of the other. The operations of mind differ
essentially from the inert properties of matter, and the
causes which induce activity in the mind, have no kind
of agency upon the physical organization of man. The
mind is governed by motives; the body is actuated
into movement by extrinsic applications.

The ancient Greek philosophers denominated the
mind *autokineton*, self-moving; and *kinetiken*, mo-
tion-giving power. They designated the body as the
organon of the *nous*, or mind; the physical medium
through which it acted. Phrenology, not satisfied with
the simplicity of this opinion, has boldly come forward
and challenged our acceptance; and in a tone of high
demand insisted, that it possesses the only key which
can unlock the mysteries of the human intellect. In a
lecture of this kind, I have not room to enter the arena
of controversy against this utopian scheme, which
sprung from the fertile region of novel doctrines, Germany, and which has been fostered in the hot-bed of all
extravagant opinions, Paris; where it is now receding
a little before the returning march of a kindred idol of
the day, animal magnetism.

The phrenologists take certain facts for granted, and
then endeavour to erect their system on such postulata.
They are not so modest as Archimedes, who asked for
a place to stand on, that he might move the world; they

assume the right to take possession of a place, though
it be in a land of shadows. They take for granted
two things, which the most acute of them cannot prove.
1st. That the faculties are instruments of the mind;
whereas the mind and its faculties are the same; what
we term a faculty being but a particular state, or mode
of operation, of the mind. For as matter, destitute of
figure, solidity, divisibility and extension, is a nonentity, so the mind aside from its faculties has no real
existence. The second position assumed is, that there
are divisions of the brain, called organs, which are to
be seen on the periphery, or surface of the brain under
the skull, which developments, or organs, impress their
figure on the cranium, or skull, in such a way as to be
noticed on its exterior configuration. Now all this
proves to be a mere matter of conjecture. Take off the
skull, and the whole surface of the brain is alike in
colour, texture and configuration; and yet we are
gravely told that the organs are there, but not to be
seen; perhaps, like the spirits in Prospero's cell, they
only come at the bidding of the master, and are "invi-
sible to every eyeball else."

Escaping from all such entangled and conjectural ex-
planations, we may adopt the opinion of the Greek
philosopher as near the truth, as the unassisted light of
nature can conduct us. It was left for a far more splen-
did manifestation of light, to clear away the obscuri-
ties which so long rested on the human mind, in reference to the nature and destiny of the spiritual principle in the bosom of man. The stream of light from
heaven which pours its full tide upon the intellect
through the clouds of our natural ignorance, has chased

away the delusions which so long cheated the human understanding under the imposing semblance of true philosophy.

It does not become us to dogmatize on a question so dark, as that involved in a view of the connection existing between the mind and the body. That there is a union of an intimate tie, admits of no dispute: that the body perishes, after a lapse of a few revolving years, we see every day realized; and that the mind will exist, independent of the body, beyond the narrow circle of time, though rationally to be inferred from the obscure glimpses of nature, is clearly announced to us by revelation.

Let us here rest satisfied, and enter directly upon the discussion of the influence of the mind in producing changes of sensation and action in the body. Coequal with the first mental emotions which we experience, is the agency which the mind exerts on the health of the animal system. Although no very urgent or lasting feelings actuate the youthful heart, yet even in the very primrose season of juvenility, the mind exerts an influence over the health of the body. Whilst the budding faculties are unfolding, and the unripened moral principles are maturing, whilst the gloss of novelty is fresh on every object around, and the song of hope enchants the youthful step—even in this period of our earthly existence, do the agitations of the passions induce dangerous attacks of disease. Thus an eminent surgeon in London tells us, that he saw the life of a fine child fall a sacrifice to the emotion of fear, induced by her school mistress shutting her up in a dark cellar. Fever, with delirium, was the consequence; during the continuance of which her constant cry was, "Don't shut me up in the cellar."

But as the powers of the animal economy grow more vigorous, and the faculties of the mind increase in strength and extent of operation, the inlets are constantly multiplying through which the impressions which minister food for thought and emotion are conveyed. As we rise higher on the scale of human existence, we tread a more elevated pathway of mental and sensitive enjoyment, and at the same time enlarge the surface upon which the impressions of pain and sorrow are inflicted. As love and hatred, grief and joy, hope and fear, by turns sway our hearts, so our bodies are affected with the alternations of depression and increased action, consequent to their variant agency. Our refined mode of life has increased in a degree beyond present enumeration the amount of painful and pleasurable sensations. Our minds are softened by the arts and accommodations of luxury, and agitated by the incessant play of those feelings which the multifarious events of life create; whilst our bodies are rendered more susceptive and excitable, from the tenderness superinduced by the soft indulgences to which civilized man is addicted.

At the same time art has multiplied her resources, and given us helps and facilities by which the evils induced by art are either prevented or repaired. Especially, has education clothed the mind with an offensive and defensive armour, by which man is enabled to wage a successful warfare against many powerful enemies. Elevated as an intellectual being, man becomes the lord of creation, and the master over the lower principles of his nature. The instinctive ferocity of the lion suffers no controlling principle of his nature to exercise a dominion over this king of beasts. But it is the glory of man, as a moral and intellectual being, to say to his passions, " Here stay thy march; and hitherto thou shalt come, but no further."

The mind of savage man approximates to the character of inferior animals. In his bosom a few strong passions have mastery. In obedience to the laws of self-preservation, he pursues the chase; in accordance with the desire of repose, he throws his body recumbent, till, awakened by the calls of hunger, or the warhoop, he rushes forwards in pursuit of his game, or dares the prowess of his enemy. His folded up powers of mind never open beneath the genial ray of education. " His intellect is not replenished; he is an animal, only sensible in the duller parts." Yet at times the *divinæ particulam auræ*, (the etherial spark derived from above,) blazes forth and enkindles the whole man.

The object of the present discussion is, not to show the effects of the passions on the language or exterior parts of the frame, these being within the appointed scope of the rhetorician and painters; but to indicate the operation of the mind, whether in its calmer exercise or more excited moods, upon the health of the animal system. Particular emotions not only have a general influence and agency on every part of the body, as an integral mass animated by the same vital laws, but a special bearing upon certain organs. Thus great anxiety of mind not only impairs the appetite, and diminishes the general vigour of the system, but often induces jaundice. This particular reference of action to an organ may depend upon an acquired or constitutional tendency to a particular disease. But when, we reflect that the converse obtains, that affections of the liver depress the mind in a singular degree, we will perceive that there is a direct, however mysterious, reciprocal influence existing between certain mental operations and different parts of the complex machinery of the human frame. Upon the fact, that the comparative development of different organs modifies the character of the individual, is built the doctrine of temperaments; a part of physiology interesting and admitting much useful reflection, but carried by some authors to an extent unwarranted by evidence.

With these general remarks, 1 will pass on to a particular analysis of the kind and extent of action excited by different emotions of the mind, on the physical structure of man.

A calm and temperate employment of the intellectual powers, will never impair the energy of the system. But a protracted and intense attention will, by interfering with the demands of the animal economy, by preventing exercise and making inroads on the nervous system, thus keeping up excessive vigilance, mar, in a considerable degree, the equable excitement of the system. Severe students are generally pale and emaciated; they have, as has been appositely said, borne the burden of lean and wasteful learning. The mind, restless by nature as the waves of Euripus, will never, under any sort of liberal cultivation, rest contented with its present images; it must have free scope in its aspirings. Those sciences which address themselves to the judgment and reasoning powers, such as mathematics, seldom injure the health, except by precluding the refec-

tion of the body from intensity of application. In large
lunatic asylums, it is very seldom seen, that a mathe-
matician has become an object of medical treatment.
For where the intellect is concerned in any pursuit or
investigation, to the exclusion of the passions, the body
will not sustain much interruption to its accustomed
health.

Poets, lovers, speculators, and all persons subject to
strong mental excitement from any urgent passion, are
the usual inmates of lunatic hospitals, in all the cases
brought on by causes, not of a physical, but moral
character. Spirituous potation, perhaps, in our country,
is a more fruitful source of that mournful wreck of the
human mind, than all the other causes combined.
Though mental occupation does not give rise to any
very formidable disease of the body, yet slight and at
times very painful affections are meliorated, suspended,
and sometimes removed, by having the mind deeply
engaged on an amusing or interesting subject. Pain in
the head is often removed by agreeably engrossing the
attention on some topic of conversation. Even fits of
the gout have been suspended by full occupation of
mind, if not unduly protracted; for gout in the predisposed is sometimes brought on by protracted mental
application, as was the case with the younger Pitt, and
with the present prime minister of England.*

When in a circle of friends, whilst the mind is pleas-
ingly entertained with a colloquial interchange of sentiment, we find that we can eat more heartily, without
inconvenience, than when our minds are not so agreea-

---

* Canning.

bly occupied. Strong mental efforts will impair, in some degree, the digestion of food, especially if the intellectual exertion be made soon after dinner; that being the chief meal, and taxing the digestive energies more than any other.

It is not, however, the act of thought which interferes with the body's health: but it is painful thinking, meditation connected with anxiety, which wears down the frail companion of the ever active spirit.

Children who have manifested a great precocity of talent, whose mind's vivacity has outrun their body's strength, seldom live long; as the adage goes, "He can't live long—he has too smart a head for such young shoulders." The cause of this issue in cases of premature expansion of intellect, arises from an undue stimulation imparted to the nervous system, and through it, as the channel of sensorial power, to the animal frame: the susceptible system yields to the overwhelm· ing urgency of the impulse thus given by the mind to the brain, and propagated from it to the various parts of the animal organization. The brain, though but an instrument of the mind, may have its chords kept in too great a state of tension, so that the soundness of that instrument is impaired.

There is a faculty of the mind of very operative and influential power, in health and in sickness; a faculty whose discursive flights at times transport the soul into elysian joys, and at other times drag it down to the gloomy Acheron. The capacity of presenting ideal scenes, of bodying the forms of things unseen, and of gilding the distant landscape of life with the brightest sunshine of bliss, is imagination. Its influence in health

9

we all experience; and its operation in disease is sig-
nally conspicuous.   It is a very prevalent opinion, that
even previous to birth, the influence of the mother's
imagination produces great effects on the child.   There
is nothing in the connexion existing between the mother and child, which would warrant us in any *a priori*
supposition, that such an event could take place.   Experience is appealed to as the decisive test, by the advocates of the opinion.   But the world is full of the
experience of prejudice.   All judgment, not grounded
on the fair exposition of evidence, is but prejudice.   To
draw sound deductions from phenomena, the mind must
be in a proper condition: it must be free from prepos-
sessions, not prone to precipitate conclusions, and disposed to examine the subject-matter in all its attitudes
and varied aspects.   It is sufficient to state, that on this
point, the experience of medical men and popular experience are antagonists of each other.—The candid
mind can determine which of the two is the best kind of
experience.

Through the potent agency of imagination, men of a
melancholy turn of mind have supposed themselves
affected with every variety of disease.   Pain is frequently fixed, and kept up in a particular part of the
body, by a concentrated attention, first awakened by
the person's imagining himself diseased in that spot.
By the powerful workings of imagination, miraculous
cures are accomplished, by what are called "faith doctors."   Quacks, and quack remedies, flourish in the
soil of a credulous public mind; and the effects of their
boasted catholicons and panaceas, are mainly ascribable
to the mystery and concealment practised; by which

the imagination is excited into extraordinary anticipa-
tions of cure. As a proof of this remark, it is well
known, that as soon as Ward's patent remedies were
revealed, by his direction in his will, they lost their reputation, which was very extensive before the composition was made known. Anthony Mesmer availed
himself of this principle of human nature, and on it
erected his system of animal magnetism. Perkins,
likewise, established his curative metallic tractors on
the same basis. Dr. Franklin, with several other members of the Academy of Sciences of Paris, were appointed to examine into the pretensions of Mesmer's
system. Franklin, from his acuteness of understanding
and philosophic power of mind, was well calculated to
detect this imposition; which the committee did detect
and expose, after a thorough examination. Mesmer
was driven in disgrace, after some considerable success
previous to the scrutiny of the committee, back to his
native fens. It is now about fifty years since he promulgated his doctrines, and after this long quiescence
in the tomb of oblivion, animal magnetism is revived
in Paris. In December, 1825, the French Royal Academy of Medicine in Paris, had an animated debate on
the question of taking up this once exploded medical
superstition, and prosecuting its investigation. This
discussion was continued to two other sittings, in January and February, 1826, it not being decided at the
first. It was decided at the last meeting, by a vote of
thirty-five to twenty-five, that a commission should be
appointed to examine animal magnetism. In this as-
sembly of the French faculty, it was stated by a member, that " he saw a woman go to sleep at the simple

will (as was asserted) of the magnetiser, who, for that purpose, was concealed in a closet of the apartment."

In a French medical journal it is stated, that, by the same art, a woman was enabled to see the time of day on a watch dial plate, though the watch was placed at the back part of the head. But the most singular effect is related by an English physician of eminence. In a visit to a female friend, the conversation turned on animal magnetism. The doctor, to ascertain the power of imagination, gravely informed her that he could practise the art. She anxiously solicited a trial of its efficacy on herself: he consented, after a little hesitation, so as to increase her desire. He made solemn gesticulations before her, passed his hand in a variety of motions around her, used some mock incantation terms; when, all of a sudden, the lady fainted and fell from her chair.

Magic, in every ignorant society of men, is the first remedy for all sorts of disease. The dominion of magic is founded in the sway that imagination exercises over the uneducated and superstitious. The father of Latin poetry has said, *felix qui potuit rerum cognoscere causas;* and the reason he gives why a man is made happy by understanding the causes of natural phenomena, is, that he escapes the enthralment of those vain fears, and superstitious interpretations of things, which the ignorant mind realizes in every event of life.

Hope is the next passion of the mind which I will notice, as having a very dominant control over the actions of animal life.

This cordial of the mind diffuses its sweetening influence through the bitterest draughts with which the cup of life is dashed. Its cheering radiance is spread over the curtained gloom of sickness. Its consolations refresh the weary spirit in the darkest period of bodily languishment. It imparts a renovating energy to the actions of the system in disease, which adds increased efficacy to the remedies administered. I cannot on this point illustrate the subject better, than by a quotation from one of the most enlightened surgeons of the present day.

"A tranquil or cheerful state of mind, (says he) under accident or disease, greatly contributes to the patient's recovery; and those who are accustomed to witness a patient in the first few hours after he has received a severe injury, auger from his manner, the probability of recovery. If he submit himself to his fate without repining, if he yield himself to the advice of his friends, and readily consents to all that is proposed for his relief, he generally does well; but if, on the contrary, he bitterly laments his fate, or his mind is actively engaged in suggesting the means of relief, impatient in their not being immediately obtained, being officious in trying to assist, anticipating every desire, such a person has a degree of constitutional irritability highly unfavourable to his recovery. It is the surgeon's duty to tranquilize the temper, to beget cheerfulness, and to impart confidence of recovery. Some medical practitioners are so cold and cheerless as to damp every hope; whilst others inspire confidence of recovery, and a disregard of situation, which supports the regular performance of all the actions necessary for restoration. It is your duty, therefore, to support hope, to preserve tranquillity, and to inspire cheerfulness, even when you are still doubtful of the issue."

To this advice of Sir Astley Cooper to his pupils, I may here remark, that my observations at the bed-side, fully confirm what he has thus judiciously suggested. It is as difficult to restore a patient, who is labouring under a dangerous attack of illness, who himself despairs of recovery, as it is to force the light of evidence into a man's mind, who has barred up the avenues of his understanding to all accession of truth, by entertaining a hatred to that evidence. To attempt the cure of a man whose mind tinges every object around with the dark colours of despair, who discredits every remedy employed, and who looks on his physician as a mere messenger of death, is like casting the ever-returning stone of Sisyphus. You may gain some temporary advantage over the disease, but even then, the despair which fills the patient's mind, puts a wrong construction on the alteration of symptoms, and those appearances which the physician hails as the harbinger of returning health, the unhappy patient looks on as the portent of his approaching fate.

But in one particular disease, hope itself becomes a most inauspicious indication. It has passed into a medical axiom, that hope springs eternal in the hectic breast. Its illusory blandishments cheat the poor consumptive patient of the misery, which might otherwise shroud his mind in the prospect of a certain death from his disease. It may have its consolations, but they are fleeting, and whilst hope fills the mind with the visions of returning health, the reality of death is not prevented. In a medical point of view, is has a very prejudicial influence, in so elating the patient with an opinion of recovery, that the means are totally neglected, or so negligently employed, at the period when they can avail any thing in arresting the progress of the malady, that unless his friends interpose and oblige him, by their entreaties, to call in medical advice, his life is inevitably consigned as a victim to the disease. Thus, with the increase of hope in direct ratio to the onward march of the disease, the mind of the unhappy individual, like the sun sinking in the western sky, when the clouds which gather round his path are illumined by his departing rays, spreads the colouring of hope over the latest hour of life; and only when life has heaved its last expiring breath, will the gay delusions of hope cease to play their part in the hectic breast.

Joy is the next emotion of mind to be contemplated in its effects on the system, in a medical point of view. In its most accumulated action, joy has extinguished life as suddenly, as could a stroke of lightning.

Pliny, says Dr. Cogan, informs us that Chilo, the Lacedemonian, died suddenly upon hearing that his son had gained a prize in the Olympic Games. Sophocles, the great tragic writer, died in consequence of a decision made in his favour, for the palm of superiority in his department of literary pursuit. Leo the tenth died of a fever, brought on by joyous agitation of mind, produced by his hearing of the capture of Milan. Hume says, that many aged people in England died suddenly of joy, upon hearing of the restoration of Charles II. The aged door keeper of Congress fell down dead, when told of the capture of Cornwallis.

Joy, when moderate, quickens the circulation, kindles up a glow of heat over the frame, and infuses strength into the limbs. Dr. Rush relates a very interesting instance of the effects of joy in contributing to the recovery from dangerous sickness: "During the time, says the Dr. I passed at a country school in Cecil county, in Maryland, I often went on a holiday with my school-mates to see an eagle's nest, upon the summit of a dead tree in the neighbourhood of the school, during the time of the incubation of that bird. The daughter of the farmer in whose field this tree stood, and with whom I became acquainted, married and settled in this city about forty years ago. In our occasional interviews, we now and then spoke of the innocent haunts and rural pleasures of our youth, and among other things of the eagle's nest in her father's field. A few years ago I was called to visit this woman, in consultation with a young physician, in the lowest stage of Typhus fever. Upon entering her room I caught her eye, and with a cheerful tone of voice, said only, "the eagle's nest." She seized me by the hand without being able to speak, and discovered strong emotions of pleasure in her countenance, probably from a sudden association of all her early domestic connexions and enjoyments with the words I had uttered. From that time she began to recover. She is now living, and seldom fails, when we meet, to salute me with the echo of " eagle's nest."

Both hope and joy are to be employed by the skilful physician in bringing about a return of health. Hope may be poured in full tide into the patient's mind, but joy must be temperately employed as a curative measure. In other words, the cheering influence of hope can never be injurious from excess of operation, but joy may overpower the frail system, and hurry the patient by a sudden stroke of mental deliquium to the grave. In hysteric and hypochondriac affections, the employ- ment of hope and joy are our principal remedies. When the mind is dejected, and the fears of the patient much excited, although his body be but little diseased, it becomes the humane physician to listen attentively to the sad tale of the patient's sufferings, and by a respectful deportment, manifest a due regard to his condition. Some unhappy individuals have been driven to madness and suicide from the unfeeling and cruel conduct of medical men under these circumstances. Whenever human misery presents itself to our notice, and implores our aid, it is our imperative duty to assist in its relief. In our efforts to impart the kindly influ- ences of hope and joy to the depressed heart, we must consult the peculiarities of the individual's mind, and external relations.—Sometimes most astonishing re- sults may flow from but a very trivial resource, where the predominant passion of the patient is brought into play, as in the following case:—Dr. Tissot relates the case of a lady in France, who could not be roused from a lethargy by any medical application, till a person, who knew the patient's love of money, put some French crowns into her hand. She soon felt the reno- vating touch of the coin, opened her eyes, and was soon restored to her reason, and bodily powers.

Love is next to be regarded by us, in its action on the health of the animal structure. Love has been divided into benevolence and personal endearment.

Benevolence diffuses a sober placidness over the frame, and is highly promotive of the healthy performances of the system.   Personal attachments are of a varied character; as the relation subsisting between the persons varies. The feelings of personal friendship are salutary in their operation. Parental love, especially in the mother, is one of the most powerful passions of our nature.   The Roman matron who died in her son's arms upon his return home from battle, after a report of his death, is a striking specimen of the overwhelming agitation it sometimes induces.

But the love between the sexes is most potent in its diversified agency on the system, of both man and woman.   Shakspeare's Viola is a good representative of what is experienced by a delicate and cultivated mind under the pent-up influence of this passion:— " She never told her love, but let concealment, like a worm in the bud, feed on her damask cheek; she pined in thought."   Man, whose mind is alternately actuated by other interfering passions, such as love of money, ambition, and love of pleasure, may escape the deteriorating influence exerted by love, not reciprocated, on the health.   When moderate love is indulged towards an object, whose heart beats in unison with the emotion thus felt; where hope can animate the mind with the prospect of a happy consummation, then, instead of impairing, it invigorates the actions of life.   But disappointed love, where the soul is " sicklied o'er with the pale cast of thought," often induces mania, consumption, and many other afflictive and dangerous diseases.

Jealousy, which results from ill-requited love, or which arises from a disingenuous disposition acting upon the passion of love, is a depressing and corroding feeling of the soul. It is a "green-ey'd monster, that makes the food it feeds on," 'and produces jaundice, dyspepsia, and infuriated melancholy.

I will next consider the most destructive passion which ever preyed upon the peace of the mind; which, in its diversified workings, produces more misery to society than all the rest, and which has more frequently quenched, with impetuous violence, the vital spark, than any other emotion.

The sententious Horace truly says,

Ira furor brevis est.
Animum rege; qui, nisi paret, imperat.

Anger is a short madness. Govern your temper; for unless you control it, it will govern you. Anger acts on the whole frame; the heart is roused into violent pulsation; the limbs are convulsively agitated, and augmented in vigour; and the nervous system vibrates with electric fire. Apoplexy often precipitates the unhappy individual into immediate death. The celebrated surgeon and anatomist, John Hunter, died under a paroxysm of anger. Hemorrhage from the lungs or stomach, from the bursting of a blood-vessel, often comes on whilst the patient is agitated by this vehement emotion. Fever frequently supervenes from the disturbance created by this passion, and gout is at times ushered in by the onset of anger. The healing powers of nature are disturbed by irritation of mind, as is illustrated by a case given by Sir A. Cooper. He was attending a man with an ulcer, which he could not heal. Several times it appeared almost well, when it

would in a little time change its healthy aspect and
grow worse.   Upon inquiry, he found the patient was
of an irritable mind, and that being in a room where
his family was, his temper was often fretted by its
arrangements. He had him removed from such sources
of angry irritation, to a distant apartment, where the
ulcer got well under the same treatment which had
failed before his removal.   The following is a melancholy exemplification of the strong dominion exercised
by anger over the mind.   A woman, says the elder
Dr. Gregory of Edinburg, whose husband had been
long absent at sea, supposing him to be dead, married
another man; but the first husband returned and
claimed his wife.   She went back to him, and after
they had lived some time happily together, she had a
child by him.   When her child was not many weeks
old, and the mother's strength imperfectly restored
after her confinement, she happened to quarrel with a
female neighbour, and a scolding match ensued; when
her antagonist insinuated that she had married her
second husband, knowing the first to be alive.   The
indignation excited by this unjust charge, brought on
an attack of mania, and sometime elapsed before she
was restored to her mind. In the mean time, her child,
given in charge to another, was shamefully neglected;
and when it was brought back to her, the shock occasioned by the change, gave rise to an immediate attack
of catalepsy.   She now became perfectly unconscious
of all around her, with her eyes fixed, her body mo-
tionless, her pulse and breathing scarcely perceptible.
In this state, if a limb were raised or extended, the muscles becoming rigid, for a short time retained it so,

until they relaxed again, and it gradually fell into its former position. The various remedies that were now employed to restore her, all proved fruitless, till it was at length deemed expedient to try what the sight of her child might do. It was brought to her, but she remained wholly regardless of it; until after repeated attempts, it was placed directly before her face, when she appeared to become sensible to it, and shortly after followed it with her eyes, and smiled, and at last stretched out her arms to receive it. When given to her, however, she pressed it to her bosom with a convulsive force, so as to endanger its life, and its removal became necessary. Mania now instantly returned, and on subsiding was succeeded by catalepsy, which alternated with each other for the space of three days, until she expired."

Fretfulness of temper is a good symptom, especially in children, after a severe attack of disease—it shows that the mind, as an embodied spirit, is realizing the union subsisting between it and the tenement of animal life, and that it is discomposed by the uneasiness resulting from the weakened energies of the body. But often, convalescence is interrupted by a fretful irritable state of mind. Especially in chronic maladies it is injurious to the patient's restoration for him to indulge in a sour, splenetic and irritable temper. Equanimity and composure conduce to the gradual return of health, in an eminent degree.

Here I may notice the effects on the health of the frame, induced by the indulgence of several comparatively minor feelings; such as malice, envy, pride and discontent.

10

The operation of these feelings is comparatively slow in the results, brought about by their indulgence, to the salutary motions of life. Malice and envy are gnawing vultures which prey with ceaseless voracity on the vitals of that man who harbours them. They create derangement of function in the stomach and liver; disturb the regular repose of the organs in sleep, and keep up an excessive action in the brain. The individual is wakeful, digests his food badly, has frequent headaches, and is generally emaciated. Pride is perhaps the father-sin of all these base feelings—for it leads a man to an excessive self-appreciation, and a proportionable depreciation of his fellow men. The proud man is apt to be malicious, envious and discontented, from the supposition that none are so meritorious as himself; and therefore that none should partake of equal advantages and blessings in human society. But as the world will not agree in this judgment of his exalted worth, he therefore becomes envious—and if any way injured or insulted, he is infuriated with revenge; and as heaven will not directly interpose on his behalf with its liberal benefactions, he is discontented with his allotment in life. In the regulations of our passions, there is none of more importance, in a medical aspect, in preventing attacks of epidemic diseases, than fortitude. Fear directly lowers the actions of life, lessens the ability of the constitution to resist disease, and sometimes of its mere agency, brings on the most dangerous maladies. The benefit of smoking tobacco, burning tar, wearing amulets and the other inert practices adopted by people to ward off the attacks of epidemic and contagious diseases, has its foundation in the confidence or fortitude which these various means inspire.

The following cases are illustrative of the dominant agency of fear on the animal economy. A man, in a London hospital, was recovering from a serious injury of one of his legs with every appearance of a speedy cure, when an ignorant pupil said, in the patient's hearing, " that leg will never get well." That day the poor fellow became feverish, his mindf oreboding a sad termination of his case; delirium supervened; the leg mortified, and in a few days he died.

A lady applied to Mr. Cline, of London, to have a tumour in her breast, cured. He advised extirpation, to which she consented with great reluctance, saying, " She was sure it would kill her." That humane and eminent surgeon assured her, that such an operation was not at all hazardous. She submitted with a calm resignation to what she said was her certain death, after having arranged her family affairs for a fatal issue—and as she predicted, so was it accomplished; she died an hour after the operation.

Dr. Wm. P. C. Barton, of Philadelphia, relates an instructive example of excessive alarm producing a state of the body, exactly simulative of the most terrific disease with which human nature is afflicted. A man was bitten by a dog, which he supposed to be mad, but which Dr. B. did not consider as affected with canine madness—under the awful fear of the approaching attack, the wretched man became miserable beyond all description. Symptoms of hydrophobia were rapidly advancing—dread of water—wakefulness—jactitation of body; and unceasing perturbation of mind. Dr. B. tried to reason with him—endeavouring to show him that the animal had not the disease—

but it was fruitless. He finally, after the poor fellow had suffered much, told him of the reputed virtues of the scutillaria or skull-cap plant, in curing canine madness. The patient caught the intelligence eagerly; Dr. B. employed the decoction of some other plant as inert as that, and his patient soon recovered.

Dr. Hamilton relates a curious instance of panic fever: A girl was taken sick in the Edinburg Magdalen Asylum, after having washed some clothes sent into the establishment from the city. The Dr. fearing contagion, had the girl's own clothes immersed in water, and her room locked up. In a day or two several more of the women sickened—their clothes were buried in water, and the house was fumigated with gas. A decided alarm now spread through the house. In four days more, twenty-two out of fifty individuals were seized with fever—some very ill, with head-ache, vomiting, &c. The minds of the most stout hearted failed: fear spread its chilling reign over the whole house.

Dr. Hamilton emancipated his mind from the delusion and thraldom of the panic—went into the sick room and in a decided tone of voice, told them it was a delusion, that they were yielding to their fears, and authoritatively bid them resume their employments. The tide soon changed, some got well that night, and in a short period of time they all recovered their health.

Anticipated attacks of periodical diseases, are prevented at times by terror. Professor Chapman used to mention a gentleman in Maryland, who cured his slaves of ague and fever, with which they were afflicted, by digging a grave and threatening the first man who had an ague, with an immediate inhumation. Terror has obliged the gouty limbed man, at times, to forego his wonted indulgence of flannel and rest, and impelled him into a sudden locomotion. Its countervailing agency has roused the hysteric and hypochondriac patients from their couch of languor and gloomy dejection, and urged them into activity and, life. But such cases are more curious than useful, serving to excite astonishment, but little calculated to direct the mind to any certain and safe practical influence.

The shock inflicted on the system by impassioned grief, has frequently snapped asunder the silken cords of vitality. In its slower operation, grief arrests the regular and equable flow of blood through the liver; produces jaundice, and infuses a torpor into the whole actions of the system. Cancer and fungus, says the high surgical authority already quoted, are frequently produced by protracted grief and anxiety. It has passed into a proverbial saying, that such a one "died of a broken heart." The heart, in its real condition, with out any figure of speech, is deeply implicated in this emotion. Diseases of that organ, as palpitations, enlargement, &c. are brought on by grief. It is apparent, that afflicted with this depressing passion, it is exceedingly difficult to restore a person labouring under any serious bodily derangement.

I have as cursorily as possible, due improvement being considered, presented to you the general and special agency of some of the most active passions on the body. You may be ready, upon a retrospect of what has been delivered, to consider that the medical poet

did not exaggerate the importance of the subject, when
he asserted that

" 'Tis the great art of life, to manage well the restless mind."

As intellectual and moral agents, who must sustain
various relative duties in society, and who must be
happy or miserable, in proportion to the discipline we
exercise over our passions, and the resources of solid
satisfaction which we find within our own minds, it is
incumbent on us to weigh well the importance of this
theme. As physicians, whose paramount duty at times
it is, to apply the soothing unction of enlivening hope
to the weary and bruised mind, under the anguish of a
pained and disordered body, we are called upon to
attend to the subject-matter of this discussion. Let us
learn from the facts disclosed above, that it should be
our great object to cultivate a mild and cheerful deportment in our intercourse with the sick. That we should
conciliate their good will, by manifesting our sympathy
for their sufferings, and whilst we remain firm in the
decisions of our judgment as regards the best plan of
restoring health, we may always let it be seen that the
hand which administers the remedy is tender, even in its
severest trials of skill. We see that the mind of a sick
person requires assiduous watchfulness, least it be in-
vaded by any of those passions which rise up in hostile
array against all our plans of extinguishing disease, and
defeat the best concerted measures which the physician
can devise.

Nothing is so well calculated to excite those depressing feelings of mind which so judiciously act on the
sick person's mind, as the injudicious visits of ignorant
and talkative people. The officious visits of well meaning but unreflecting persons, do the sick incalculable

injury. Tedious tales and idle gossipings, disturb the repose so essential to the sick. Sometimes persons are so forward as to interfere in the prescriptions of the physician, or so exceedingly imprudent as to suggest doubts as to the skill of the medical attendant, even in the presence of the individual oppressed with disease and great mental inquietude. Such conduct is reprehensible in the extreme; if such persons wish to suggest any thing, it should be done to the friends alone. Discreet friends are of great service by infusing the cordial of social sympathy into the sick man's bosom. Physicians are sometimes taxed with being enemies to religion, because they oppose the promiscuous intercourse of religious persons with their patients. Perhaps, at times, physicians are too tenacious on this point. They forget the constitution of the human mind, and overlook the importance of the soul. But, let there be here a fair estimate made of the difficulty and delicacy of accomplishing the object in view, that of soothing the harassed and dejected mind of the patient, without too great a danger of sacrificing his life. Let there be a liberal interchange of sentiment on this point, between physician and the clergyman or religious friend. It is of great importance at times, that the patient should have his mind rendered calm by religious communication. That physician who refuses to grant his patient an opportunity of having his oppressed heart relieved of its burden, by the cheering irradiations of religion, is contending against even the temporal good of the sick man. Of how much greater importance are the interests of eternity, let the man who has darted an anxious eye beyond the present scene of things, determine.

LECTURE

ON THE RESPONSIBILITIES OF THE MEDICAL PRO-
FESSION; DELIVERED IN THE LOUISVILLE
HOSPITAL, AUG. 27, 1831.

GENTLEMEN:

In bringing the series of summer lectures, to which
you have so attentively listened, to a close, I cannot
take my leave of you, in the capacity of an humble
contributor to your improvement in medical knowledge, without dwelling, for a few moments, on the
responsibilities involved in the practice of the profession which you have adopted for your pursuit in life.
The dignity and importance of the medical profession,
are to be correctly estimated by a due consideration of
the great and responsible duties devolving on physi-
eiaus in the exercise of their vocation. It is a work of
magnitude that you have undertaken. High and difficult are the intellectual and moral efforts demanded,
that you may attain the great ends of the profession.
In order to fill your minds with a just appreciation of
the extent, variety and greatness of the obligations
which are connected with the profession of medicine,
advert with serious attention to the leading scope and
ultimate aim of all medical knowledge. The physician
operates not on brute, unconscious matter. His sphere

of agency brings him in direct contact with life—the life of his fellow men. He holds in his hands the earthly destiny of his fellow beings; to him is committed the awful and responsible task of watching over, with scientific eye, the workings of disease as they prey on the health of fathers, mothers, children; and of either, by his skill, restoring them to the cheerful light of day, or, by his ignorance, hastening them into the darkness of a premature grave. I am aware that medicine, in its best estate, is an imperfect art; that even when its most faithful and skilful ministers have availed themselves of all the resources of the art of healing, they have, in many instances, to lament the limitation of their means of cure. Still, much good can be accomplished by a scientific application of those remedial powers which a kind Providence has placed in the hands of man. Disease may be arrested in its ravages on the human frame—pain alleviated, or subdued, and life made more tolerable, even under incurable maladies, by the judicious prescriptions of the skilful physician. My object, gentlemen, in this lecture, is not to throw a grain of incense on the altar of professional vanity—not to magnify the men who practise medicine, but to magnify the office of a physician, by indicating some of the more prominent duties devolving on medical men in the exercise of their professional functions. I wish you to feel the great and responsible position you are at a future day to occupy in society, and to impress upon your minds the moral necessity which is laid upon you of making due preparation for your contemplated sphere of life. Let the importance of the station be rather felt and acknowledged in its beneficial results, than ostentatiously displayed by any course of offensive conduct. Then the consciousness of the magnitude of your undertaking, instead of being suffered to evaporate in vain airs and pompous pretensions, will produce a concentration of your powers in the exertions you employ to prepare yourselves for an honourable discharge of the duties of the profession. You should apply to the work with zeal, and anticipate important results. The moment you think lightly of your profession, your resolutions abate, and imbecility and relaxation of effort take possession of the entire man. No man ever excelled in any profession to which he did not feel an attachment bordering on enthusiasm. A high and honourable feeling of emulation should breathe through all your studies. This feeling is the plastic spirit which, penetrating the depth of your souls, rouses every energy of your moral and intellectual being to run with usefulness and renown the race set before you. Permit me to remind you that the chief distinction and crowning glory of man, is his intellectual and moral nature. That the developments of this intellectual and moral nature, are the ultimate purpose of all education. That the active faculties of the mind, and the best feelings of the heart, are never more powerfully elicited than when brought to bear in the exercise of the high functions appertaining to that active occupation of life which you have chosen. And think not that I utter language, on this occasion, at war with sober reality. The estimate put upon the medical profession by the brightest intellects is in accordance with the above declaration. Let me adduce the testimony of one or two disinterested witnesses. The celebrated poet, Pope, thus speaks of the members of our profession: "They are, in general," says he, "the most amiable companions and the best friends, as well as the most learned men, I know." The learned Dr. Parr, of England, asserts, "That after a long and attentive survey of literary characters,- I hold physicians to be the most enlightened professional persons in the whole circle of human arts and sciences." Blackstone, in the introduction to his Commentaries, advises physicians to read law, in order "to complete the character of general and extensive knowledge which this profession, beyond all others, has remarkably deserved." I have sheltered myself behind the above eminent authorities to sustain me in the high appreciation which I have put upon our profession. The demands made on the intellectual and moral capacities of the physician, are full of solemn responsibility. Diversified and accurate knowledge on all the branches of the science is, of course, of indispensable importance in order to qualify him to practise the art of curing diseases with success. But the physician should not only be learned in medical science—intimately conversant with the structure of the human body, and possessed of a comprehensive acquaintance with the principles of medicine—but he must be an honest man. Not merely honest in his pecuniary transactions; but honest in a higher and more extensive sense. He must possess the *to kalon* of character; he should be a man of honourable, liberal and noble bearing in society.

The science of medicine is a vast field of investigation; and the practice of it is a thorny and perilous

way, in which a stern trial is made of moral integrity.
To the study of the science, you should bring faculties
disciplined by a previous training of classical instruc-
tion, and of the other branches of a liberal education.
Your minds should be qualified, by previous habits of
study, to undergo a protracted process of analysis, of
deduction, and of research. If your mental powers
have not been exercised in intellectual inquiries before
you commence the study of the science of medicine,
you will be liable to be discouraged by the first difficulties which present themselves, and abandon the toil-
some task altogether, or irritated into impatience, your
minds will be driven to the more objectionable plan of
creeping along the path thus beset with obstacles, with
discredit to yourselves and injury to society. The great
fault of the young men of our country is an unwise and
restless desire prematurely to enter upon the scenes of
active life—whence results a crude and superficial preparation for the responsible duties of the respective
professions they follow. This evil does not exist to the
same extent, nor has it so injurious an influence on
society, in the mechanical avocations as in the professions of divinity, law and medicine. A young man is
generally obliged, by the articles of his apprenticeship,
to undergo a proper novitiate that he may be qualified
to be a good workman. I am aware the different religious denominations of our country are every day becoming more and more convinced of the demands of
society for an enlightened ministry. Legislative enact-
ments guard the bar, in some measure, from the incur-
sions of ignorant lawyers. And, in some of the States
of our Union, there are severe laws against quackery in

medicine. Still, especially in Kentucky, the profession of medicine is overrun with greedy and rapacious followers of mammon, who care neither for the honour and dignity of the healing art, nor for the lives of a credulous public who employ them.

Gentlemen, truth has its sternness and authority— and it obliges me thus to speak.

The consequences of this eager and impatient wish to rush, without due preparation, upon the arena of active life, sheds a fatal blight and withering spell upon the future eminence of every young man who is under its governing authority.

The late Judge Tilghman, of Pennsylvania, in his eulogy on Dr. Caspar Wistar, who was one of the most distinguished supports and ornaments of our profession, very justly observes, "It has been remarked that, with few exceptions, those who have been great in the learned professions, have abstained from practice at an early age. The cause is obvious. The elements of science lie too deep to be attained without long and patient thought. The mind requires retirement and tranquillity, to exert its powers of reflection to their full extent. But these are incompatible with the bustle, the anxiety, the agitation of active life." When a young man precipitately throws himself forward in the ranks of an active medical career, he soon feels his inadequateness to the office he has thus most unwisely— nay, most iniquitously undertaken. Finding that he cannot sustain himself by the internal resources of his own mind, and not having moral honesty enough to resist the allurements of gain, he has recourse to the various shifts, crooked ways, and degrading expedients,

by which quackery seeks to entangle its victims.   Or,
if his remaining feelings of pride will not allow him to
practise the arts and devices of the nostrum vender, he
still is apt to slide into a sort of vapouring, or assume
eccentricities of conduct, alike inconsistent with real
science and the honour of a high-minded man.

Dr. Rush; who has written with so much ability on
the ethics of the profession, and who has reflected such
a flood of light on practical medicine, makes the following judicious remarks on that spirit of empiricism which
so much disgraces many of the professed members of
the faculty. ·

"There is," says Rush, "more than one way of
playing the quack.   It is not necessary, for this purpose, that a man should advertise his skill, or his cures,
or that he should mount a phæton, and display his dex-
terity in operating to an ignorant and gaping multitude.
A physician acts the same part in a different way, who
assumes the character of a madman or brute in his manners, or who conceals his fallibility by an affected gravity, or taciturnity in his intercourse with his patients.
Both characters, like the quack, impose on the public.
It is true, they deceive different ranks of people; but
we must recollect there are two kinds of vulgar, viz.
the rich and the poor, and that the rich vulgar are often
on a footing with the poor, in ignorance and credulity."

· You thus perceive, from the language just quoted
from the greatest medical philosopher America has
ever produced, that, for a physician "to advertise his
skill or his cures," is placing himself side by side with
him who pretends to cure disease with a secret remedy.
The principle involved is the same in both cases.

Both characters attempt to impose upon the public by holding out false allurements to confidence, and, by a crafty appeal to ignorance and credulity, strive to win a spurious reputation. The true dignity and honour of our science, demand of every physician who regards his profession with any elevated conceptions of its rank and of its utility, to frown upon every man who thus attempts to impose on the public. Each enlightened and honourable medical man is bound by the highest considerations of the duty he owes himself and of the responsible relations he sustains to the profession and to the public, to employ every moral resource in his power to repress the spirit and exercise of quackery in medicine. There are men who make the profession of medicine a base medium through which they can practise, successfully and with impunity, delusion and imposture; and who, governed by sordid self-interest, creep their reptile way along a filthy path, to the summit of public confidence—whose best acquirement is that of a bold asseveration of the cures they *intend to perform,* and of whom it may be said, that the only benevolence they manifest, is that of giving a quietus to the troubles of their patients, by a speedy dismissal from life. The nostrum vender, or dealer in secret remedies, daily and hourly contravenes the obvious philanthropy of our profession, in wrapping up in impenetrable mystery and secrecy, for bis personal profit, those means of restoring health which, in his venal dissimulation, he pretends to possess. The great ornaments of medicine have been men of the warmest benevolence—whilst empirical pretenders have ever, Cacus like, concealed their remedial agents in the gloom of a depraved selfishness. Jenner, the illustrious benefactor of his race, was a type of the true physician. Bombastus Paracelsus was the representative of the vampyre brood of quack doctors. '

Medicine is a liberal and intellectual pursuit. All mystery and concealment are in direct opposition to the spirit of our science, both in its intellectual and moral bearings and tendencies. " Come and see" is the inscription which blazes in living capitals on the front of the temple of medical science. This noble edifice stands with its foundations built on the rock of truth; its portals are open day and night, for the admission of every sincere inquirer after knowledge, and on the walls within are hung the votive tablets of the many thousands who have been cured by the faithful ministers that trim its golden lamps, and burn sacred incense on its altars. Without its hallowed enclosure are seen the base tribe of greedy quacks, and venal pretenders, who ply their lying trade about its walls, and seek protection under the shadow of its ample dimensions.

To every true disciple of the healing art is committed a high and responsible trust of keeping the deposit of his profession's honour with untiring watchfulness. To such belongs the delicate, and, at the same time, magnanimous office of watching over the best interests of the profession. That physician proves derelict to his duty, who is found mingling in the ranks of the nostrum monger and prating mountebanks of the profession. What! shall the educated physician be seen associating on terms of professional equality with him who practises artifice and imposture, in order to circumvent and delude a credulous community? Shall those who have gathered their inspiration and their light from the high priests of our science, pollute themselves by such disparaging intercourse? Must we countenance those who *call themselves* physicians,

> " As nimble jugglers that deceive the eye,
> Drug-working sorcerers that change the mind,
> Disguised cheaters, prating mountebanks," '

to play off their cozenage on the people, without any disapprobation on the part of enlightened and virtuous physicians? Shall a degrading rivalry in money making, extinguish the light of all honourable feeling in the minds of medical men? Let each young man who beholds such a disgraceful exhibition, as is sometimes seen, of successful charlatanry, rest assured that the reign of error and imposture is brief—that the foundation of the empiric is laid on perishable materials, and that, though he may amass wealth, no sure and abiding honour attends his career. Veracity is violated by such a man every time he administers his nostrum, for he is practically setting his seal to a delusion which his own false statements have engendered? Is truth, the tutelary genius of science, the best friend of erring man, and the only sure guide and safeguard of our happiness? Then, the man who wilfully propaga es a lie and practically affirms it, is, most assuredly, the enemy of his race. The nostrum - vender is, therefore, an enemy of man; he is a blot and an anamoly on the beauteous face of God's moral creation, and should be shunned as the upas tree—for he lives in an atmosphere of deception, delusion, imposture, and sordid self-interest.

The responsibilities of the medical man are of a momentous kind. He is to understand his profession well, before he attempts to practise it; and he is bound, by every just consideration of his responsibleness, to improve himself every day, in order to meet the daily demands made on his skill with augmented usefulness to society. Gathering, from every available quarter, the elements of knowledge, he must, by intellectual analysis, convert them into the sound deductions of a well balanced judgment. But he is called upon likewise to be a man of strict veracity, of exemplary sobriety, and of faithfulness to his professional obligations. Truth should be personified, as it were, and put into unceasing exercise by the physician. He should reject all ostentation and paradeful exhibition of his business, and manifest a dignified simplicity in his intercourse with society. A man, filled with a desire to fulfil his duty, lives for reality, and not for display. The ways of duty to such a man are direct, and the means of accomplishing them simple. Such a one has intellectual and moral improvement always before him, and, regulated by this unity of view, he preserves habits of candour and honesty with himself and with those around. Cultivate, therefore, this true dignity of character, and, let others debase themselves as they may, ever preserve this moral excellence. Animated by these views and considerations, your course will be onward and upward; step by step, you will ascend into a freer atmosphere, and reach a more expanded pros-pect. Thus all your energies will be borne along unconditionally and unreservedly towards the objects to which you should consecrate yourselves with absolute devotedness. Let every thing be consistent in your plan; then there will arise no embarrassment in the execution of the work undertaken—your minds being fixed in a just decision, and your efforts springing from a determination to achieve the object before you.

Let the crafty empiric boast of his success in a course of sordid and groveling self-interest, in which career he has sported with the credulity and ignorance of the multitude. But remember that the only stable success attends the men whose intentions are honourable and upright. Such men, by degrees, are discovered and made known; they form immutable and advantageous connexions with society, and their reputations are guarded by a deep-founded esteem, which is increased and confirmed every day. Disdain mean, transient and little ends, and seek a wide and solid foundation for your professional standing. Rise above the mere motive of accumulating money, to the kindling energy and solemn joy which are inspired by an enlarged philanthropy. Fear not to oppose popular delusion when it bows down at the footstool of charlatanry; nor ever hold intercourse, or in any other way give encouragement to men who are " cheating the eye" of the public " with blear illusion," in order to make that illusion the pander to their base desire of personal aggrandizement.

In conclusion, let me press upon your consideration, the necessity of a calm and determined perseverance in the pursuit of professional eminence. Remember that weakness of character is restless, impatient, and full of contrariety of purposes—that a feverish and imaginative mind, which is ever changing its plans of action, can never arrive at any elevation; that fixedness of purpose is absolutely essential to success in any laudable enterprise, and that no man can excel in any walk of life, unless he has power to adhere to the motives which first suggested his determinations. The world, it has been truly said, is full of people who have conceived and undertaken great and noble things, but who failed in their accomplishment. Perhaps there are very few well regulated minds, who have entered upon the investigation of medical science, that did not form some brilliant plans of professional eminence, and hoped to realize them. But how soon the efforts of many quail before the difficulties of the way; how very few reach the bright goal which once glittered before their aspiring wishes! How melancholy is it to see the ocean of life covered with so many wrecks of lofty hopes and noble aspirations! But, gentlemen, I hope better things of you. Your career, I trust, will be one of usefulness in the world. May you have patience to labour with sedulity of endeavour in the profession which you have adopted, and may a hallowed feeling of benevolence actuate your minds in diffusing around your path in life the fruits of that charity which is " twice blessed" —blessed in him who gives, by irradiating his soul with the peaceful smiles of an approving conscience, and in him who receives, by smoothing the brow of anguish, and restoring health to the pained and diseased body. Then your course will be luminous, with a divine radiance, and " the blessings of them who were ready to perish" will descend on your heads, fraught with the purest joys which man is allowed to taste in the present introductory stage of his immortal existence.

INDUCED BY MERCURY.

My design in the following observations is, 1st, to institute an inquiry into the mode by which mercury acts upon the system;—in the 2d place, to point out the causes of its morbid agency, and in the last place, to particularize the most common forms of disease engendered by it, and their most appropriate means of treatment.

There is no article in the whole compass of our remedial resources which can at all be compared to mercury in the extent, power and diversity of its modes of action on the system. Nor is there one which, in the hands of a judicious practitioner, can be made to wield such an ascendant influence on the deranged functions of life, and on the structural lesions which often impend the organs, as the different preparations of this mineral. In its crude state, as quicksilver, it possesses no appreciable power, when employed as a remedy, except that resulting from its great specific gravity. Contráry to the assertion of Pliny, Galen, Hippocrates and Dioscorides, and of even some of the earlier modern writers on this subject, fluid mercury, when free from alloy, exerts no deadly property at all;

nor does it exert any positive agency by its direct contact with the living surface of the stomach and intestines, as large quantities have been repeatedly swallowed without injury. Gaspard shut up large quantities of quicksilver in the various cavities of the body without observing any other result than that arising from the irritation of a foreign body. To remove obstinate constipation, fluid mercury was formerly a fashionable remedy; but it is now entirely abandoned, from several well authenticated cases of rupture of the bowels being induced by its mechanical force. Fluid mercury, at the ordinary temperature of the atmosphere, discharges copious vapours. These vapours will rapidly mercurialize the persons who inhale them. Two well known instances of most violent salivation being induced in the whole of a ship's crew by the exhalations from a large quantity of quicksilver, were witnessed in 1810, on board the British ships Triumph and Phipps. Every person on these vessels was more or less affected by the mercurial vapours, and all the cats, dogs, sheep and goats on board were destroyed. The bags containing the mercury, which had been rescued from the wreck of a ship near Cadiz, soon burst, after being stowed in the holds of the respective ships, and the metal lay in the bottom of the vessels, in a mass.

The accumulation of an amalgam of tin and quicksilver in the cells of the colon may be the occasion of great inconvenience, and of ultimate death. Such an instance came under my notice in 1821, in Louisville, Ky. the place of my former residence. A Mr. Prior, a merchant of that city, had for many years been tormented by the presence of a tape worm in his alimentary canal,

and for the expulsion of which many remedies had
been ineffectually employed. In accordance with Dar-
win's suggestion, a respectable and enlightened physician
directed him to take the amalgam of tin filings and
mercury. The remedy was taken agreeably to the following directions. Twelve ounces of tin and an equal
quantity of mercury were mixed together, and divided
into twenty-four parts—one of these doses—of an ounce
each—was to be taken every hour till the whole was
swallowed. Fifteen ounces were taken during the first
day, and the day subsequent, according to directions,
he took a saline purgative, which operated well, and
brought away near forty feet of tape worm, with a small
quantity of the amalgam. Subsequently Mr. Prior took
four more ounces, making in all nineteen ounces taken;
and he felt confident, when I saw him in the winter
of 1821, that of this quantity at least sixteen ounces remained in his bowels. Upon examination, and being a
very thin man, the examination was very satisfactory,
the amalgam felt as large as a hen's egg, and was lying
about mid way between the umbilicus and the superior
anterior spinous process of the ileum, being quite
moveable, and producing on pressure no pain. Whenever he rode on horseback priapism was quickly induced,
and he wore a belt around his abdomen to keep the
mass more steady in walking. He took this amalgam
in January 1820, and it remained permanently lodged
in the colon till his death, which took place in 1822.
Being attacked in that summer with slight fever, inflammation, ending in gangrene, soon arose in the intestines. Upon post mortem inspection, it was found
that the portion of bowel in which it was deposited,

had sloughed before death. The amalgam was preserved with a portion of the intestine, by Dr. Galt the attending physician. Mercury, when subjected to trituration with unctious and other substances, such as chalk, manna, conserve of roses, &c. is reduced to the condition of an oxide, and in that state acts on the organic sensibility. The only preparations in ordinary medical use are the ointment, the red precipitate, the blue pill, the hydrarg. cum creta, the bichloride or corrosive sublimate, and the protochloride or calomel. The sulphurets of mercury, like the metal, according to Christison, are not possessed of any deleterious action on the animal body. Of mercurial compounds the red precipitate and turpith mineral act as irritants, and possess the common property of all the compounds of the mineral, of creating mercurial action on the system. Corrosive sublimate is a potent irritant and poison, so are also the nitrates of mercury. The cyanide or prussiate of mercury is analogous to corrosive sublimate in its deleterious agency on the body. Calomel is the most valuable of all the forms in which mercury can be administered. It is more extensively used than any other mercurial preparation, and from its facility of exhibition, has inflicted more mischief from an abuse of its powers, than all the other mercurial remedies.

The specific irritation and corrosive effects of the corr. sublimate are so well known that it is not proper to dwell on them. The only sure antidote to the poisonous agency of the corrosive sublimate is the white of eggs. Thenard, the eminent chemist, several years ago, by mistake, swallowed a mouthful of the concentrated solution of corrosive sublimate for water, and was saved by Orfila's discovery. The white of eggs was quickly taken, and he suffered no harm. Several years ago I was called to a negro man who had taken a considerable quantity of corrosive sublimate to destroy his life, because his master refused to sell him to a gentleman he was very desirous of living with. There being a dozen of eggs in the house, he was made to swallow the white of every egg—and the antidote was entirely successful.

In considering the agency of mercury on the animal body, I shall inquire into the local action of the different mercurial preparations, and in consecutive order investigate their constitutional effects. Given in minute doses, corrosive sublimate acts as an alterative, with especial reference to the skin; but in quantities over a half a grain, it ordinarily acts as an irritant. Used as an escarotic, it often effects much good, in stimulating diseased parts into recuperative efforts which terminate in their cure. But it should be employed with much caution as an external remedy, for death has often resulted from an incautious use of it, either in powder, solution, or ointment, when applied to ulcers or eruptions of the surface. Intense salivation, sometimes accompanied with symptoms of gastric irritation of a violent kind, follows its application occasionally to wounds or eruptions. In the London Medical Repository, vol. 16th, a case is given of death following the application of a solution of corrosive sublimate to an eruption on the scalp of a child—great ptyalism ensued, which destroyed the patient in a few days. I was taken to see a gentleman in 1819, when residing in Louisville, who was then in a state of great salivation from

12

the action of a nostrum, applied at least eight months before my visit, to a fungus cerebri. - This gentleman had sustained an injury on the top of his head, which produced after some months a diseased state of the bone, as well as of the dura mater. The external tumour was extirpated by the knife, but there ensued a rapid destruction of the bone, and finally a fungus cerebri. A Dutch quack, who had gained celebrity for curing ulcers by a secret remedy, was employed, after the failure of repeated excisions with the knife, and of pressure, to stop the growth of the fungus. His nostrum was a strong solution of corrosive sublimate, with the addition of a drachm of borax to every four ounces. This he applied every day till a most copious salivation ensued—and then the remedy was abandoned. The case proved fatal, several weeks after my visit.

The local action of the mild mercurials, claims our especial consideration. In what manner does calomel or blue pill influence the vital operations of the stomach and intestines? The French physicians generally regard calomel as an irritant, and therefore highly improper in all cases, when any degree of gastro-enterite is suspected. But in what way do they arrive at this conclusion? First, by most dogmatically pronouncing on the action of the remedy, and then they resolutely reject its employment. And this in the open sunlight of a counter practice, distinguished for safety and wisdom. Circumscribed within the narrow enclosure of a most abject dread of its powers, they pertinaciously and superstitiously abhor the use of calomel. To the credit of a few able French physicians, let it be added that calomel is not thus treated with unmerited contempt.

Baudelocque, in his work on Puerperal Peritonitis, has lavished much praise on mercury; as the surest remedy in that fatal malady. Is calomel an irritant, when applied to an ulcer on the cornea? To talk of irritation being created by it in such a case, is to use words without logical accuracy. " Those," says Sir W. Philip, " who are prepossessed against it and other powerful medicines, in their fear of the medicine are too apt to lose the fear of the disease." Mr. Annesley, in his " Practical Observations on the Effects of Calomel on the Mucous Surface and Secretions of the Alimentary Canal," has detailed several experiments on dogs, to show that calomel, even in large doses, " has the effect of diminishing vascular action, rather than of exciting it; which will account, in some degree, for the scruple-doses of calomel at once allaying irritability of stomach and vomiting—a circumstance I have witnessed with astonishment, and for which, I never could account till now. These experiments were followed up by the performance of others, and the results were always the same. I am led, therefore," continues he, " to the following inferences, the former of which is confirmed by Dr. Yelloly's interesting paper on the vascular appearance of the human stomach, read to the Medico-Chirurgical Society, July 27th, 1813—that the natural and healthy state of the stomach and intestinal canal is high vascularity; and that the operation of calomel in large doses is directly the reverse of inflammatory." In fever, when the stomach is so irritable as at times to preclude the use of any other internal remedy, calomel given in minute doses every hour, will often, nay, generally, subdue the vomiting, and restore calmness to the distressed organ. 1 had two very alarming cases of bilious colic, several years ago, which occurred in my practice, close to each other, in which one-grain doses of calomel, in pills, given every half hour, was the remedy that saved life in both cases. One patient was bled, and blistered on the abdomen, but still the vomiting was incessant. The other was a delicate female, whose pulse would not admit of vascular depletion. In both cases, obstinate constipation was present, which enemeta did not at all relieve. Each was directed to take one grain of calomel every half hour. The man whom I had bled, becoming impatient, took the medicine more rapidly, pretending that he had lost the pills. In the space of twenty-four hours, the lady had taken forty-eight grains, and the man in thirty-six hours took more than one hundred. The vomiting continued with little or no abatement, in each case, till the gums became sore, and then ceased with the spasmodic pain of the bowels, which were easily acted on afterwards by oil. Here every circumstance was unfavourable to an absorption of the mercury, for the stomach constantly rejected it, and not enough was retained to act on the bowels, and yet ptyalism ensued; and in both patients was quite urgent in two days after the medicine was discontinued. Here, says the Broussaist, is gastro-enterite, or simple gastritis; and will you give so perturbating a medicine as calomel in such a case! Is medicine a practical art, and are we to arrive at its facts by the inductive method of philosophizing? If so, try the remedy ere you condemn it—yes, try it faithfully in our bilious fevers, especially of the West and South, and then, and not till then, are you competent to pass a judgment on the merits of the practice recommended above. Calomel, blue-pill, and the hydrargum-cum-creta, when given as aperients or purgatives, in ordinary cases, do not act as irritants. On the contrary, no milder medicines can, in numberless instances, be given, particularly in the intestinal disorders incident to deranged hepatic function. No cathartic can be selected from the materia medica which operates so kindly upon infants as calomel. Not that I would carry its administration as far as a practitioner in Louisville did in his own infant's case; but I would not be deterred by an unfounded figment of its perturbating quality to use it, as I have done during nearly twenty years, discriminatively, according to the emergent demand. The physician referred to above, gave his child, an infant of less than a week old, within two days, near one hundred grains of calomel, and it recovered of the attack of intestinal irritation under which it was labouring. Calomel when given in immense quantities, will often pass through the intestinal tube, unchanged. I saw it evacuated in small masses, with little or no discolouration, in the case of a gentleman, who was taking thirty grains every two hours. There are three successive stages in the phenomena which arise in the stomach, intestines and collatitious viscera, after calomel is received into the alimentary canal.* The first stage is that of decomposition of the calomel to an oxide, of a dark gray colour; without which operation of the living surface and its secreted juices on the calomel, it will exert no subsequent action on the alimentary tube. The second result developed,

* Annesley.

12 *

is the stimulus, peculiar and unique, exerted by the
calomel upon the mucous tissue of the stomach and
bowels, by which a change is wrought in the secretory
action of that tissue.   The third effect is the excitement
imparted by the remedy to the bilious and pancreatic
secretions, augmenting or altering them.   The unrival-
ed power of calomel in dysentery, is abundantly confirmed by the valuable experience of James Johnson,
Annesley, Ainslie, Musgrave and others.   Dr. Ainslie
prefers small doses, but the weight of authority is in
favour of the large doses indicated by Johnson, and in
which he is followed by Annesley and Musgrave. The
increased secretory action created by calomel on the
surface of the intestinal canal, and on the pancreas and
liver, is generally imparted to the kidneys and skin; so
that after the cathartic operation of calomel, or blue-
pill, these several emunctories are in a more vigorous
discharge of their offices than anterior to the agency of
the remedy.

There are two constitutional ways in which mercury
acts.   The first is a more alterant and tranquil action;
and the second is accompanied by more potent demonstrations of the powerful agency of the mineral. Dr.
W. Philip has written a very good essay on the influence of minute doses of mercury, in which he strenuously insists on the beneficial effects of giving the
remedy in very small quantities, persisting in its use
for a long time.   He contends that it possesses a twofold property of stimulation and sedation, and that to
effect these ends, it must enter the blood.   Since the
day of Cullen, who denominated mercury a stimulant
to every living fibre, when constitutionally acting,

almost every writer on the subject has concurred with that great man in his views of its action. There are two leading and prominent points now to be noticed, which lie before our way of investigation, and must be distinctly elucidated before any just conceptions can be entertained on the modus operandi of mercury on the body. The first point is embraced in this question, is mercury a stimulant? The second point is embraced in another question—does mercury enter the blood?

If mercury is a stimulant, in what sense is it one? for it is clear upon the most superficial consideration, that it does not incite, or goad on the actions of life in any manner analogous to camphor, or volatile alkali. Then if really a stimulant, in what manner or degree does it excite the functions of life? If authority were of itself sufficient to settle such a controverted matter as that involved in the modus agendi of mercury, then there would be no room for further remark. For the preponderance of medical opinion is greatly in favour of the stimulant operation of mercury on the constitutional energies and actions. Thus Ainslie says, "Mercury, I conceive to be the most universal stimulant and alterative in the whole range of the materia medica."[*] And in this view he has the concurrence of Hamilton, Alley, Eberle, and others. Dr. Chapman says, "though undoubtedly a stimulant, and of the most enduring kind, its effects, I think, cannot be ascribed to this property simply." John Hunter considers it a stimulant, and that it destroys the "diseased action of the living parts, counteracting the venereal irritation by produ-

* Materia Indica, vol. I. p. 648.

cing another of a different kind," and that, therefore, "neither quantity alone, nor evacuation, will avail much; but that it will be quantity joined with sensible effects that will produce the quickest cure, which from experience we find to be the case."*

There are several very important respects in which, if mercury be a stimulant, it differs from all other articles of that class of remedies. First, other stimulants are withheld by the enlightened practitioner in conducting the treatment of diseases of acknowledged inflammatory character. Take, as examples, dysentery, acute hepititis, iritis, puerperal peritonitis:—to administer brandy, camphor, or any other stimulant for the cure of these diseases, would be a strong evidence of dementation. And yet mercury is the sheet anchor of the treatment in such diseases.

In the second place, mercury refuses to act when the system is too much prostrated in its powers. But stimulants are always given when the vital energies are sunk, for the purpose of increasing them. Sir W. Philip, aware of these wide points of dissimilarity in the action of mercury, and of any stimulant article, properly so designated, contends that " mercury, like other agents, possesses the sedative as well as the stimulant property:—and its sedative property appears to be wholly exerted on the motive powers—for when it appears to lessen the sensibility, this effect seems to arise from its removing some cause of irritation." Now such an explanation is neither precise nor profound. "Like other agents, mercury possesses the sedative as well as the stimulant property;" then it, and all other

* Hunter on Venereal, p. 320. 1st Am. ed.

remedies act in the same way—and the question is un-resolved, in what does the agency of mercury differ from that of other remedial articles. There is still another aspect in which the distinctive character of mercury is to be contemplated, as regards its action on the animal body. It possesses a cumulative property, different from all purely stimulant articles, bearing an analogy in this respect to arsenic and digitalis. To secure and perpetuate the train of action created by stimulants, we have to increase the quantity adminis-tered, and often to change the agent, because the im-pression induced by them upon the organic sensibility, is constantly diminishing. It is otherwise with mer-curial excitement : to continue the remedy in a less dose than the one you commenced with, after the pro-cess of mercurialism is instituted, is to greatly enhance the effect. The period which sometimes elapses be-tween the administration of mercury and the develop-ment of the salivant effects of the remedy is often considerable. In this a wide difference is seen between its action and that of any agent belonging to the class of stimulants. Swediaur, in his work on venereal, men-tions a case in which the mercurial action did not break forth till more than a month after the use of the mineral. Dr. Hamilton, in his work on mercury, gives the fol-lowing as as instance of the cumulative property of mercury. "A lady, the mother of four children, in the twenty-eight year of her age, had a bad miscarriage at the end of the fourth month. When the author was called, she was very much reduced from the loss of blood, and required the ordinary palliative remedies. Three days after the first visit, she complained of a bad taste in her mouth, with soreness of her gums, and on the following day salivation took place. On inquiring into the circumstances of her previous history, it was learned, that four years before, she had had for a fortnight a course of blue pill, which had only slightly touched the gums, and it was solemnly asserted, that she had never again taken any preparation of mercury, and had been in general good health. The salivation, with the usual consequences of emaciation, debility, and irritability, continued for above twelve months. Occasionally for a day or two it was checked, but alarming vomiting, with threatening sinking of the living powers, supervened. The patient, however, eventually recovered. The medicines administered, during her illness from the abortion, were carefully analyzed, from a suspicion that some mercurial preparation might have been mixed with them, but it turned out that they contained no mercury."

Dr. Ives, in a note, gives another case derived from J. M. Smith, M. D. immediately in connexion with Dr. Hamilton's, at p. 23 of Ives' Ed. of Hamilton on Mercury.

"In November, 1811, says Dr. Smith, I was requested to visit a lady about 55 years of age. Her symptoms were small and frequent pulse, tongue white with a brownish discolouration through the middle, protracted constipation of bowels, hot skin, head ache, delirium, and great prostration of strength After premising purgative medicines which effectually relaxed the bowels without mitigating the febrile symptoms, I put her on the use of submuriate of mercury, combined with pulvis antimonialis and opium. This preparation, containing about two grains of the submuriate in a dose, was repeated every three or four hours with the design of exciting ptyalism. This plan of treatment was continued three or four days, with the occasional administration of other remedies as the circumstances of the case seemed to require. At the expiration of this period, symptoms of ptyalism not being manifested, and the patient rapidly sinking into typhus, I was induced to abandon the mercurial treatment, and to pursue a more stimulant course; accordingly I advised the liberal use of wine and other cordial remedies. The good effects of this plan were soon discernible. In a short time she became convalescent, and in a few weeks was able to leave her apartment and visit abroad.

"Three months after her first attack, I was again desired to see her. She exhibited at this time all the violence of mercurial salivation, and, with much difficulty related the manner of its accession. Three days before, after considerable exposure to humidity and cold, she observed her breath to smell disagreeably, and the saliva to flow copiously. Fœtor of breath increased to that degree that she avoided company, fearing her presence would be offensive. At the same time her gums became sore and tumid, and at length ulcerous; the tongue was swoln and loaded with much white mucus, and excessively sensible; the salivary glands, generally, were also affected with intumescence: indeed, so severely was she affected that she had scarcely the power of utterance. So correspondent were her symptoms with those which mercury is known to occasion, that I did not hesitate recognising her present illness as the effect of that medicine. Not suspecting at this time

that the affection of her mouth was produced by mercury received into the system at a period so long previous as when she laboured under typhus, I made spe
cial inquiry whether she had recently taken any medicine, and was answered in the negative, and informed,
that she had taken nothing of a medicinal nature, since
she was under my direction while sick with fever. Not
doubting her veracity, and being persuaded that her
disease was a mercurial ptyalism, I was led to inquire
to what source it could be attributed. While engaged
in this inquiry, her former illness occurred to me, and
the quantity of calomel taken at that time without producing any sensible effects. To account for the disease
from this source appeared to be deviating from correct
etiological reasoning, yet so decidedly marked was her
disease, that I felt no hesitation in assigning this as the
cause. For her relief I prescribed the occasional use of
flowers of sulphur and cream of tartar, with a view to
keep the bowels in a soluble state; and dirceted the
mouth to be frequently washed with a detergent gargle:
under this treatment she soon recovered a state of perfeet health." This suspended cumulative property of
mercury I have often witnessed, to a limited extent, in
fever. Very frequently after the employment of calomel for a number of days in febrile diseases, without
any appreciable manifestation of mecurialism in the
system, a very noticeable subsidence of the worse features of the attack would be witnessed, and *pari passu*
with the patient's improvement, would be the outward
signs of the mercurial action. The secret springs of the
disease had been touched by the remedy before the
external phenomena, attesting its pervading operation

in the system, had revealed themselves. For a change in the series of morbid actions going on in the organs is a surer evidence of the remedial control exerted by the mercury than fœtor of the breath, and swollen gums. The return of salivation after a lapse of some time, I have seen in several well marked instances. In a boy of six years old who had been badly salivated during an attack of bilious fever there was for several, winters a recurrence of foul breath, swollen gums, and ulcerations about the mouth. The mercurial erethysm returned, after exposure to a cold and damp air. Fever always accompanied the recurrence of the mercurialism. The question whether mercurial action is susceptible of a complete intermission, formed a material subject of inquiry, in a criminal prosecution some years ago, in England. A woman was indicted for murdering her master, by giving him corrosive sublimate. He had been salivated two months previous to the severe salivation which terminated his life, and the question was whether this last salivation could be attributed to the mercury taken before, after so long an interval. The medical witnesses were in direct opposition to each other in their statements. The surgeons of Lock Hospital deposed that such a thing as an entire intermission of salivation from mercury was seen in the wards of that institution—that in one case the interval was three months, and that in one patient there was a periodical attack of salivation at intervals of a month or six weeks for a whole year.*

Dr. Gordon Smith in his Principles of Forensic Medi-

---

*Christison on Poisons, 2d ed. p. 372.

cine cites from Dr. Hamilton's lectures a case in which the interval was four months.

From the foregoing facts and reflections it must appear evident that mercury is not a stimulant—if we appropriate that term exclusively to such medicinal agents as increase the vital powers and actions, without inducing any sensible evacuation. Stimulants impart force and activity to the movements of life; and rouse the whole economy into a more vigorous performance of its functions. But mercury accomplishes no such end by any direct bearing and operation—that it quickens the circulation and increases secretory effort are no proofs of its being a stimulant, for great depression of the motive powers, and prostration of nervous energy are too often seen during its sway over the functions, to warrant any sound inference that it is stimulant because it thus affects the heart and the emunctories. It is sufficient for all the purposes of practical medicine, to determine what the phenomena are, and the order of their development, which we observe in the living body whilst under the dominion of mercury. It is alien from the spirit of just philosophy and adverse to the acquisition of a true experience of the benefits to be derived from the employment of mercury, to classify such a remedy, acting, as it does, with a unique and most exclusive agency, with any other remedial substances. It stands alone, insulated in its own wonderful and extensive capabilities of good or evil, and in solitary strength bids defiance at all our weak attempts to compare its properties with any other article in the materia medica.

Have we any well authenticated, incontestible proofs

that mercury **ever énters** the blood? A hundred tongues and pens are ready to enter the arena of controversy at once, and with precipitate zeal, put down all doubt or dispute on the point. And the attenuated form of the antiquarian and bibliomaniac, covered with the dust and cobwebs of his closet, is seen gliding with rapid strides across the arena, ready to throw at our heads the large tomes of Brasavolus, Rudius, Schenkius, Poterius, Hochstetter and other most illustrious cultivators of hypothetical illusions. But let us hear what they say for themselves in this matter. "Bonetus," says a late writer, "gives us séveral instances, collected from Renodœus, who states from Trajanus, hydrargyrus copiosus repertus est, in *cranio* nempe, *scapularum* at *brachiorum* juncturis."

Cardanus took two ounces of crude mercury out of a patient of his own—which he no doubt had put there *after* death. Schenkius saw a patient vomit a spoonful of quicksilver, during a mercurial course. Rhodius saw two patients piss crude mercury; and in the German Ephemeres, says Christison, it is said, that no less than a pound of it was found in the brain, and two ounces in the skull-cap of one who had been long salivated!! Buchner avers, that Pickel of Würszburg obtained mercury by the destructive distillation of the brain of a venereal patient, who had long taken corrosive sublimate. This same Buchner detected abundance of quicksilver in the blood, in the saliva, and urine of mercurialized patients. Now, says the humoralist, with the pride of certain victory sparkling in his eye, what can you say to these stubborn facts. If the facts are not stubborn, they are at least amazing and miraculous. **For as the** moderns, with the best improvements in chemistry, can make no such discoveries, or rather inventions, we must rather presume, with some of the former very erudite disciples of Galen, that the human body has undergone a change in its anatomical structure, than that Pickel or Schenkius could misinterpret or misrepresent facts in an age of wonderment and superstition. All that I shall pointedly urge *in answer* to the above is by way of illustration. " Dr. Cooke mentions a case, says Professor Christison, in which the fluid in the ventricles of the brain had the smell and taste of gin, the liquor which had been taken.* It is added that the liquid was inflammable. It would have been desirable that Dr. Cooke, or rather his informer, Sir A. Carlisle, had mentioned how the inflammability was proved; for some fallacy may be strongly suspected; because gin of sufficient strength to take fire, could not enter the blood-vessels without coagulating the blood, and so preventing its further progress." In addition to the above, the same author states, that in animals poisoned with alcohol introduced into the stomach, he never could perceive even the smell of the spirits in any other part of the body.†

John Hunter, Philip Syng Physick, Bostock, Christison, with many of the other acute and herculean minds of the profession in modern days, have never been able to detect mercury in the blood, saliva and bones, in the manner, *it is said,* the wonder-loving explorers in this dark mine of inquiry, in former ages, found so readily and in such abundance.

* Cooke on Nervous Diseases, p. 104, Am. Ed.
† Christison on Poisons, 2d Ed. p. 802.

"Mercury," says the great and original man, who stands as the father of modern English surgery, "often produces pains like those of rheumatism, and also nodes which are of a scrofulous nature; from thence it has been accused of affecting the bones, 'lurking in them,' as authors have expressed it. It may be supposed to be unnecessary to mention in the present state of our knowledge, that it never gets into the bones in the form of a metal, although this has been asserted by men of eminence and authority in the profession; and even the dissections of dead bodies have been brought in proof of it; but my experience in anatomy has convinced me that such appearances never occur. Those authors have been quoted by others; imaginary cases of disease have been increased; the credulous and ignorant practitioner misled, and patients rendered miserable."*

Dr. Physick, in the fifth volume of the New York Medical Repository, has given the result of his experimental investigation on this subject. "So confident," says he, "were they formerly of mercury entering the system, that it was even believed, in some instances, to have been deposited in the bones in the form of quicksilver. The latter opinion has been sufficiently disproved by accurate anatomical investigations; though the former continues still in vogue, and is generally believed." In that communication, the Doctor relates some experiments performed by himself and Dr. Seybert, upon the blood and saliva of patients, affected with mercurial salivation, and then adds, "The introduction

---

* Hunter on Venereal, p. 316.

13 *

of mercury into the blood-vessels through the absorbents, (an hypothesis which appears to have been admitted by physicians without much examination) is at least rendered very improbable by the above experiments. It may, indeed, be said, that the mercury is combined with the blood in such a peculiar way, that the above means have not been adapted to detect it; but such an objection must be granted to be a very lame one, because it is hypothetical."

Mayer, not long ago, subjected to accurate chemical analysis, the chief solids and fluids of a person who died while taking mercury, and Devergie, so late as 1828, by a very delicate process, so delicate as to enable him to detect a 122.680th part of corrosive sublimate in blood, endeavoured to detect mercury in the blood, saliva and urine of persons under a mercurial course: and Christison tried to find mercury in the solids and fluids of two rabbits killed by inunction, but the result in all their hands was, that no mercury could be found.

Dr. Bostock states, in his "Observations on the Saliva, during the action of Mercury on the System," that he could not detect the minutest portion of mercury in the saliva of a patient deeply affected, both locally and constitutionally, with that agent. "We learn," says he, "from the experiments, in the first place that no portion of the mercury is actually present in the fluid, from which it follows that the effects of this medicine, although so remarkably manifested on the salivary glands, must be produced through the medium of the system generally, and hence we may presume that all the organs destined for the secretion of mucus will undergo the same change. This change would appear to consist essentially in the conversion of the animal matter, from the state of mucus to that of a serous, or rather of an albuminous fluid.* ·

Mercury sometimes produces fatal effects in very small quantities. Dr. Ramsbotham, in the first volume of the London Medical Gazette, gives a case of fatal salivation from fifteen grains of blue pill, taken in three doses, one every night. Dr. Crampton, in the fourth volume of the Transactions of the Dublin College of Physicians, relates an instance in which two grains of calomel, caused ptyalism, extensive ulceration of the throat, exfoliation of the lower jaw, and death. Three drachms of mercurial ointment employed in the way of inunction have induced violent salivation and death in eight days.†

Dr. Hamilton gives a case in which five grains of blue pill, given within three nights, created such an intense degree of sialagogue effect, that for a month the lady's life was in the utmost jeopardy.

Dr. Alley, in his work on Hydrargyria, relates the case of Francis Milroy, aged ten years, to whom only three grains of calomel as a purgative were given, in whom it produced a severe eruption over the entire surface of the body.

In persons who have been severely ptyalized, I have seen a single grain of calomel, or a few grains of blue pill renew, after a lapse of months, a painful degree of salivation.

How can these facts, and those before cited in refer-ference to the suspended cumulative action of mercury,

* London Medico-Chirurgical Transactions, vol. 13th, p. 79.
† Christison.

and the intermissions often observed in mercurialism
of the system, with the crude and absurd notion of the
introduction of mercury into the blood? During the
days of medical superstition, when every sort of idle
tale concerning the effects of medicines was credited, it
might answer very well, as a substitute for knowledge,
to talk about venereal poison floating in the blood, and
tell the credulous that mercury had a specific elective
affinity upon such virus to neutralize and expel it. But
now when the phenomena of disease are studied, as
they are seen, in the living solids, and when with such
a mass of contradictions and errors darkly rising before
our view on the whole field of humoral pathology, it
behoves every one who desires to talk sense, and adhere
to things open to examination, no longer to indulge in
the fond vagaries of a wandering and excursive fancy.
If mercury enters the blood in one patient it should do
so in every one, to whom it is given to an extent sufficient to salivate.   If it does so in every case why did
not Physick, Seybert, Bostock, Christison, Mayer,
Devergie, and many other acute experimental inquirers
detect it, assisted, as they were, by the lights of modern
chemistry? Besides, mercury will not act as a salivant
on many constitutions.   In one case I gave it in large
quantities for a number of days without witnessing the
smallest manifestation of ptyalism. The gentleman had
venereal, and was otherwise in good health.   If it enters the blood, why did it not affect the system as a
sialagogue in this case? It did not purge my patient, or
to any great extent, act on any of the emunctories. Let
us recur to the question, how does mercury act? First,
it acts as a purgative locally on the stomach and intes-

tinal canal. Secondly, its action is radiated to the pancreatic and hepatic functions. Thirdly, its circle of operation is more widely diffused in its agency on the kidneys and skin, and still more expansively directed to the glandular apparatus of the mouth. Not that the action of mercury is invariably, in all states of the system, precisely in this consecutive order of influence. But when it is judiciously administered, its range of action is as indicated. There is an additional capability of impression upon the constitution which seems almost peculiar to this sovereign remedy. That capability resides in its governing influence over the diseased movements of the capillary system in many cases of disordered health. Dr. Farre, in view of this power of arresting the inflammatory process in iritis, contends that mercury has the power of preventing or arresting the deposition of coagulable lymph. "I have uniformly regarded," he writes to his friend Mr. Travers, "the mercurial action as the most effective means of arresting the disorganizing process of adhesive inflammation, whether of the iris, or of any other texture of the body."*

Arsenic acts on the capillary system, particularly of the skin, in a most effective manner in many diseases. But mercury has a more penetrating and dominant control over the capillary system than arsenic. This is strikingly evinced in fevers of a low grade, termed by Armstrong congestive, where the skin is cold and bloodless—directly the mercurial impression is created on the constitution, the surface becomes warm, and as-

---

* Cooper and Travers' Surgical Essays, art. Iritis.

sumes its functional action. The increased action of the heart, consequent on mercurialism, results from this development of energy in the capillary system. In this sense is mercury a stimulant, but if regarded in other lights, it is the very opposite of a stimulus. Its agency is a peculiar, mixed, characteristic one—totally unlike that of any mere stimulant, or sedative, or evacuant, or of all combined. By the union of no other remedies can you imitate, with any success, the widely diffused operation of mercury on the constitution. When given in very small doses it produces a slow and permanent change in the deranged condition of the functions. And yet with all its capability of restoring health to the organs, and of preventing or arresting morbid depositions of lymph, mercury is often a most potent engine of mischief. My next object is to point out the causes of its evil effects upon the living animal body. The first cause which produces the morbid affections springing from the agency of mercury on the system is idiosyncrasy. An inscrutable peculiarity of constitution renders it a matter of great peril for some persons to take mercury in any shape. The smallest dose of blue pill, or calomel, will in such individuals create the most alarming symptoms, and death will sometimes result from the taking of a few grains of either. Sir W. Philip mentions the case of a lady in whom salivation was caused by one fourth of a grain of blue pill; and in another lady's case, one grain of calomel equally distributed in eighty pills of extract of liquorice was prescribed—one pill to be taken at a time—but that the 80th part of the grain of calomel so affected her with depression and irritation, as to compel the abandonment of the remedy. In the summer of 1822, I attended a lady with violent dysentery, in whose case a few grains of calomel produced the most intense degree of erethismus—death seemed to impend each time she took the remedy. And yet in consultation it was determined to persevere in the use of the remedy, as it appeared the only resource left us for her restoration. The dose was increased from a few to ten grains every four hours, and under this treatment she recovered. This idiosyncrasy obtains in certain persons in relation to the agency of other articles, both dietetic and medicinal. Opium is like poison to some constitutions, even in the smallest quantity.

The second cause operating in the production of the morbid consequences arising from the administration of mercury is the inapposite condition of the system at the period of its being given. Thus a broken down constitution cannot bear the mercurial action. If the vital forces are either in a very exalted, or depressed state, the administration of the remedy to produce a constitutional effect, is injurious. The strumous diathesis, is well known to be unfavourable to the beneficial agency of mercury. Neither young children, nor aged people, can withstand a powerful mercurial impression. Another cause which is frequently the origin of the mischiefs inflicted by the action of mercury on the body, is the excessive quantity administered. That there is a point of limitation as regards the quantity of calomel to be given, is quite apparent, not only because the practice of medicine requires judgment to discriminate in reference to each case of disease, how far a remedy may itself become an evil, but on account of the subaction, that calomel must undergo in the stomach, before it will influence the organic sensibility of the mucous tissue of the bowels. It is not desirable, by any means to throw into the stomach, a substance which will lie there as a mechanical weight. To give therefore an ounce, or half an ounce of calomel, in one dose; as has been done, is a practice unwarranted by sound therapeutical considerations. Fifteen, twenty, or thirty grains of calomel are as large a dose as any exigency would seem to demand. Ten or twenty grains of the remedy repeated twice, thrice, or four times a day, is as far as the practitioner should proceed in cases requiring the medicine, unless the stomach rejects it soon after being administered. Where the physician desires to induce, rapidly, the constitutional result of mercury, in addition to the use of calomel, he should sedulously employ inunction, or the dressing of blistered surfaces with the ointment. That the reader may judge of the extent to which the practice of giving large doses of calomel has been carried in this country, the following is copied from Dr. Cooke's Remarks on Cholera, as it appeared in Lexington, in June, 1823. In " case 6th," of " A. Walker, a man of 40, perhaps," who called at the professor's house, "and complained of uneasiness in his bowels, but there was neither vomiting nor looseness. His complexion was very bilious." Sixty grains of calomel were ordered, at 12 o'clock in the day time, he took the dose, and at night it was repeated; second day an ounce of calomel was given, and tincture of aloes; third day, " he took more calomel, in similar doses"—we infer of an ounce each, and died on the fourth day.

"Case 7." A black woman took two ounces, in two successive days, and recovered.

"Case 9." A coloured girl of ten years of age, "took half an ounce of calomel, and repeated it several times in the course of a few days." She got well.

"Even a table-spoonful," says Dr. Cooke, "did not always effect the object"—that of producing bilious discharges from the bowels. "A black girl at Mr. Benjamin Theiser's, took several such docs before the watery discharges were stopped. Bilious discharges then followed, and tincture of aloes, about a wine-glass full at a time, kept them up, and she recovered."

" Case 26. William Douglass," rested satisfied with "taking twenty grains of calomel early in the day," of his illness. Dr. C. gave him a table-spoonful of calomel in the evening of the same day. Next morning early, another table-spoonful of calomel was given," and continuing to live, contrary to all expectation, and the discharges continuing the same, he took the same quantity (a table-spoonful) every six hours on that day, and the next, and the third."* The young man died, the Doctor thinks in consequence of bad nursing, and a change in the form of the aloetic medicine. In consultation with a physician who held views similar to the author just quoted, it was proposed by him to administer to a man very ill with cholera, an ounce of calomel—half immediately and the balance in half an hour, or an hour, " in order," says he, with great apparent consciousness of the perspicacity of his supe-

---

* Transylvania Journal of Medicine, for July, August and September, 1834.

rior judgment, "to tap the liver, and make the bile run freely." He declared that he would have nothing further to do with the case, unless his prescription was followed; and as the other medical men, with myself, took another view of the propriety of thus tapping the liver, the heroic doctor retired from the field, in perfeet disgust at the timidity of the other less knowing ones.

A still additional cause, which often operates in producing disease and suffering of a most protracted kind, thus inflicting on the patient an existence which is loathsome and torturing in the extreme, is improper regimen, or a reckless exposure to the vicissitudes of atmospheric temperature, during a mercurial course.

In warm climates, in which a uniform temperature is maintained, the ill effects arising from a sudden arrest given the functions of the skin, whilst the system is under mercurialism, are seldom experienced. But even in India, according to Ainslie, pernicious effects flow from the use, or rather abuse of the remedy. "The Hindoos," he remarks, "reckon mercury one of their most powerful medicines, but are very apt, not always intentionally, to induce, by its use, the most frightful salivations; I say frightful, for however desirable it may be that the mouth should be touched before we can be certain of much lasting good having been done, few things are more distressing than severe ptyalism."* Musgrave, who practised in Antigua, observes, in his essay "On the unmixed Effects of Mercury on the System," that he never saw or heard "of a case where

* Materia Indica, vol. II. p. 349.

symptoms bearing the stamp of secondary syphilis, in the common acceptation of these words, were ever suspected to be the offspring of mercury administered for the cure of any other disease"—that the only bones he ever saw immediately or ultimately affected by the most aggravated cases of mercurial mismanagement, were those of the upper and lower jaw, whose vitality might have been partially destroyed by a process of denudation, caused by the extensive sloughing within the mouth, which involved their periosteum."* It is a well known truth among practical physicians, that to conduct with skill, a mercurial course, strict attention should be paid to the condition of the patient's system. If he lives on in the indulgence of stimulating food, partaking perhaps of wine or spirits every day, he incurs great hazard of injury to his constitution, from the exorbitant or perverted actions created in the organs by the mercury. And when we reflect upon the great powers of the remedy, as evinced by the processes of functional activity which it arouses in the system, no surprise should be excited at the great evils resulting from the reckless manner with which patients often conduct themselves during its administration. Subsequent reflections will be offered on this point, as the discussion is proceeded in.

But in verity, and without misconception, is there any such thing as mercurial disease at all, or is it a mere nonentity, the "the shadow of a dream," infesting the brains of the ultra anti-mercurialists? It would have been well for many an unfortunate patient had mercury been

* Edinburgh Med. and Surg. Journal, vol. XXVIII. p. 54.

fraught with no properties but those which are saluti-
ferous—were it *never* the dire messenger of evil to the
suffering human being who has been tormented by its
potent sway. And although Carmichael of Dublin,
very high surgical authority it is readily conceded,
avers that he had not, " nor did he believe that any
other person had witnessed ulcers on the skin and
throat, and nodes on the bones, from the exhibition of
the most-extensive courses of mercury in any other
than the venereal disease, nor even an eruption, except
the well known mercurial eczema,"* yet Mathias,
'and other medical writers, most positively pronounce
the contrary to be the fact. And my own limited experience in this matter has most impressively taught
me, how much easier it is to dogmatize than to prove,
in reference to the position taken by Carmichael. Mercury may produce disease by its direct immediate action on the stomach, or surface—or it may induce its
morbid effects by a slower operation through the general system. By its rapid irritating impression on the
gastric mucous tissue, or upon the skin, it may act as a
poison, either from idiosyncrasy of the constitution, or
from some peculiar condition of the nervous system.
The instances already cited show that mercury sometimes acts as a violent irritant, and Pearson in his "Observations on the Effects of various Articles of the
Materia Medica in the cure of Lues Venerea," in speaking of the erethismus mercuriale which affected some
of his patients, observes that, by abandoning the mercury for a few days or weeks in the cases of patients

* Ed. Med. and Sug. Journal, Vol. XI. p. 436.

thus affected by it, he always found that he afterwards
could with safety return to its use, without the individuals experiencing any bad consequences from its
administration.. In its quick action on the first passages the mildest preparation of the mineral may bring
on, 1st, Emesis and vomiting. In the second place the
genuine erethismus mercuriale may result;—or, in the
third place, a vesicular eruption may be developed;—or,
in the fourth place, the patient may be affected with a
very severe, perhaps dangerous, inflammation of the
throat and mouth. When the constitutional influence
of mercury is exercised, disease may result either from
the excess of the action instituted by the remedy, or
from that influence being checked, thwarted or interfered with, by exposure, to a cold and humid atmosphere, or by improprieties of living. In the constitutional class of cases we have ulcerations of the skin and
throat, pains simulative of rheumatism, nodes, and
sometimes destructive inflammation in the nasal car
tilages.

- The severe emetic quality sometimes evinced by calomel is generally owing to a peculiar susceptibility of
the individual, whom it thus affects. I have never
known any bad result arise from the emetic or cathartic
operation of calomel, though Hoffman tells us of cases
of death from the violent operation of the medicine on
the first passages. Trotter, in his Nervous Temperament, has related some cases to show the dangers incur-
red by the free use of calomel; but he seems to labour
under a nervousness himself on this point, and practically illustrates, in his horror of mercurial remedies,
the doctrines of his book on such nervous maladies.

Erethismus mercuriale was first accurately described by
Pearson in his Observations on the Effects of various
articles of the Materia Medica in the cure of Lues
Venerea. He thus describes it:—" Erethismus mercuriale is characterized by great depression of strength, a
sense of anxiety about the pœcordia, irregular action of
the heart, frequent sighing, trembling, partial or universal, a small, quick, and sometimes an intermitting
pulse, occasional vomiting, a pale contracted countenance, a sense of coldness; but the tongue is seldom
furred, nor are the vital or natural functions much disordered. *

The vesicular eruption, termed by Pearson, eczema
mercuriale, or rash from the use of mercury, denominated by Alley hydrargyria, and by Spens and M'Mul-
len erythema mercuriale, and by Moriarty mercurial
lepra, is sometimes occasioned by a single dose of calomel, or a small quantity of mercurial ointment rubbed
on the thighs.

The *Tremblement Mercuriel*, or Shaking Palsy,
may likewise be induced by the sudden impression of
mercury on the system—it is rarely the result of the
medicinal use of the mineral; but most always arises
from the inhalation of mercurial vapours, by miners,
gilders, barometer makers, and glass platers.   Dr. Dar-
wall says that he once " saw the tremour established in
a child, to whom a considerable quantity of calomel
had been given for incipient symptoms of hydrocepha-
lus."†

* P. 156.

† London Cyclopedia of Practical Medicine, Vol. 1, p. 152.

"On the whole," says Christison, "those who are liable to the shaking palsy do not appear liable to salivation. Even those who undergo mercurial frictions may have it, according to Mérat: and M. Colson, who confirms this statement, quotes Swediaur as another authority for it. It is not merely long-continued exposure to mercurial preparations that causes the shaking palsy; a single strong exposure may be sufficient; and the same exposure may cause tremours in one and salivation in another. My friend Mr. Haidinger, the mineralogist, has mentioned to me an accident a barometer maker of his acquaintance met with, which illustrates both of these statements. This man and one of his workmen were exposed one night, during sleep, to the vapours of mercury from a pot on a stove, in which a fire had been accidentally kindled. They were both most severely affected, the latter with salivation, which caused the loss of all his teeth, the former with shaking palsy, which lasted his whole life."

The attack of mercurial palsy is sometimes, though not often, sudden, but most commonly it comes on gradually; at first with defective control over the muscles of the arms, followed by slight convulsive snatches, and agitations which terminate at length in a tremulous state, increasing in intensity, and extending to the legs, and whole body, if the patient continue his exposure to the cause. The accompanying symptoms of the trembling are arid and unhealthy brown skin, distended belly, and generally a slow pulse; the appetite and digestion are generally good, and sleep sound. A single dose of calomel will sometimes occasion severe and long continued salivation. In the summer of 1814, whilst a student of medicine, I saw a coloured woman severely ptyalized by five grains of calomel given at night; the salivation came on before morning, and continued distressing for a week.

Dr. Christison mentions the case of a chimney sweeper, who died in consequence of gangrene of the mouth produced by cleaning a gilder's chimney, during which operation he felt a disagreeable sense of tightness in the throat.

In the summer of 1821, I attended with Dr. G. W. Smith, the patients of a temporary small hospital in Louisville, Ky. which had been opened by the citizens for the poor of the town: the present commodious edifice, erected by the state for a marine hospital, was not then built; neither was there an alms house, which now exists. There were carried to this house a woman and child, both very ill. The child was six years old, and had been sick with fever before admission. Whilst at home, five days previously, it had taken six grains of calomel, agreeably to a physician's order. The physician directed the mother, for she was at that time able to attend to her child, to give it as much cold water as it wanted. Soon after taking the calomel, and subsequently, it drank copiously of cold water just from the well. In a few days, no other medicine being given, its mouth became sore, the mother being too sick to attend to it, the poor thing was neglected. On the fifth day a small black spot appeared externally on the cheek, and the internal surface of the cheeks was discoloured, the lips were swoln and puffy, and a most unpleasant odour affected the breath. On this day the child and mother were admitted into the hospital. The

mortification of the cheeks was unchecked by any remedy, and complete sphacelus of the whole left cheek
taking place in two days after its admission; it soon
died. The cold water in this case unquestionably caused
the mischief which arose.

I have seen another case, which happened in the
practice of a respectable physician of Louisville, in
which the child took several doses of calomel, before
the mouth became inflamed, and the patient was saved
with the loss of nearly all the teeth in both jaws, and a
portion of one cheek—about half an inch from the left
corner of the mouth having sloughed off. A blister was
applied to the cheek, in which the red spot, the fore-
runner of the gangrene, made its appearance: charcoal
powder was freely used to correct the fœtor, the temperature of the skin was kept up by warm clothing,
and the bowels were kept open with sulphur and charcoal; the child being sustained by small quantities, frequently given, of well-made chicken soup.

In the spring of 1815, whilst a student of medicine,
a case of great interest came frequently under my notice. It was the case of a young man who, having contracted the venereal disease, applied to a learned, but
very negligent, practitioner for the cure of it. He was
put under a course of mercury without any preparation,
or discipline. He ate, drank, and exercised as he was
accustomed to; and during the course he slept in a cold
room, in the winter season, drank iced water in the
night when thirsty, and sleeping near a window with
a pane of glass out, he was exposed to a current of the
cold air on his head. In a short time his throat became
sore, and severe pains affected his joints. All this was

nothing, but the poison of Venus traversing his veins—
as he thought, and as, perhaps, his physician learnedly
communicated to him.   The calomel, and inunction,
were now plied with more assiduity and earnestness to
overtake the virus, with which his blood was so replete.   But he had became worse—severe pains seized
his head, nodes made their appearance on his bones,
and ulcers commenced on his scrotum and dorsum
penis. Thus beset and distressed, he abandoned his physician and applied to the medical man, with whom I
was studying.   His case proved a most intractable one,
and often did he declare that were it not for the dark
mystery of the future, to him one of peril and dread,
that he would abandon life by an act of self violence, so
full of bitter suffering and wretchedness were his days.
Cicuta, Lisbon diet drink, and similar remedies were
tried with little advantage.   Neither arsenic, nor powdered sarsaparilla were employed in his case.   After a
few months he went to New Orleans, and there his
health improved gradually;   but he has since informed
me that he was finally cured by boiling down two gal-
lons of water, into which half a pound of gum guiacum,
broken into small pieces, had been put, into a gallon,
and taking a quart of this every day.

About twenty years ago there practised a physician
in a part of Kentucky, who as familiarly dealt out calomel by the spoonful, as Broussais does his ice water. The
result of this practice was mournful in the extreme, according to the declaration made to me by persons in
whom reliance could be placed.   In one family several
children were deformed about the face, in consequence
of the sloughing induced in the lips and cheeks, by the

enormous doses of calomel given, for even ordinary attacks of fever.

The following cases are given as examples of mercucurial disease, as springing from the excessive or perverted action of the medicine.

In the summer of 1826, I attended a stout young man with slight fever, accompanied, however, with great cerebral disturbance. He was bled repeatedly, and actively purged by mercurial, and other cathartics. Contrary to directions, he used cold water, both externally to his head, and as a drink. His mouth becoming slightly sore from the frequent doses of calomel which he had taken, the cautionary precepts respecting the use of cold water were reiterated. Whilst his mouth was sore from the mercurial influence, he would persist in washing his head all over with the cold water. He recovered and went home to his farm, a few miles from Louisville. Before his system had entirely recovered from the mercurialism, he exposed himself on the farm, going through the fields, whilst the grass was wet with dew, and lying on the green sward in front of his house, during the early part of the night. In about five or six weeks, subsequent to his departure from town, he called on me with rheumatism, or an affection in his knees and ancles, very similar to the chronic form of rheumatism. I gave him some medicines, which he did not take very faithfully. In the course of a week or ten days, eruptions came out on his skin, in different parts of the surface. They were of a copper-colour, not painful to any considerable degree, and which had simultaneously appeared with tumours on the shin-bones, and on the radius of the right arm. He grew worse, his throat became inflamed and suppurated, and he was unable to walk, from several ulcers on the thighs and legs. I prescribed arsenic internally, and directed him to wash his ulcers with diluted nitric acid, holding opium in solution. But this lotion irritated his sores, and aggravated his sufferings. He quit me, and applied to a country practitioner, who discontinued my remedies, although he concurred in my opinion of the nature of the disease. He now took small portions of sulphur to neutralize the mercury in the blood and bones, and washed the ulcerations with the solution of sugar of lead. The patient grew worse under this plan of treatment, and again sent for me. I found him, after a lapse of several weeks from my last visit, with very bad ulcers, superficial and spreading, on the thighs, arms and back. A dense scab, in the process of the sore, was first formed, and the ulceration commenced under it. In this way, originated the phagedemic ulcers, which were rapidly forming in different parts of the body. He was now ordered to resume Fowler's solution of arsenic, fifteen drops, three times a day, to be gradually increased to thirty drops, in a tea-spoonful of tinct. guaiac. ammon., to be taken in a cup of milk. His ulcers were dressed with the common saturnine ointment of the Dispensatory. After persevering in this treatment six or seven weeks, his ulcers healed up, and the nodes disappeared; but there remained a slight efflorescence on the forehead. His strength was so well repaired, that in the end of November, he went fox-hunting, and afterwards on the same day, being Sunday, sat in a country church without fire;—the day was damp, windy and cold for the season. In a day or two after this last exposure he was seized with an excruciating affection of the scalp, and pain and swelling denotive of periostitis in the lower end of the radius of the right arm. . There was no reappearance of the eruption. By my advice he was bled several times, and took Dover's powder, at night, to, enable him to sleep. The bleedings rather aggravated his sufferings, but the anodyne produced alleviation of the pain and procured repose. Subsequent to this, he took an emetic of ipecacuanha every other day, which produced pretty full vomiting. His diet was milk and mush, or bread. The repeated emetics conjoined with Lisbon diet drink, and small doses of antimonial wine, on the intermediate days, restored him to tolerable state of health, but there remained some lameness of the left knee, which was swoln and stiff. This young man afterwards visited the southern part of Kentucky, and remained in sufficient health to travel to St. Louis, in Missouri. In going to the latter place, he was exposed to the rain, and by the time he reached his place of destination, he was again affected with pains and stiffness of the joints, sore throat and cutaneous eruptions. He called in a physician at St. Louis, who upon hearing a history of his case, promptly and unhesitatingly pronounced it to be syphilitic. . In vain the young man protested that he never had any sore on the penis, nor had he ever exposed himself to the infection. That made no sort of difference, was the doctor's reply, he might have caught the disease on the seat of a privy, or by sleeping in sheets in which a man with the venereal had lain all night, and the matter might so secretly insinuate itself into his blood, as that he might be utterly uncon-

15

scious of the time and mode of its ingress. So positive
was the medical man on this head, and so confident in
his averment of rapidly and permanently curing him,
that he persuaded him to submit to a severe mercurial
course at once.   This was in the month of May, 1827.
Large doses of calomel were administered to him,
which rapidly and most severely salivated him, with
an aggravation of all the symptoms.   With difficulty
he reached Louisville in a steamboat.   Upon his arrival,
he commenced taking Swaim's nostrum, but finding no
benefit from its use, again sent for me.   By the arsenic
and tinct. guiac. he regained, during the summer, his
health.   In 1828 he had, apparently, entirely recovered
from the effects of the mercurial disease; and he got
married and settled in town.   But upon getting very
wet, when heated at a fire, he relapsed.   After several
months he again was restored to some degree of health,
until winter, when he grew worse.   I lost sight of the
case till January, 1830, when I was requested by a
respectable physician to see him in consultation with
him;—he had salivated him for lues venerea, but with
most evident injury.   I saw him but once, for we could
not agree in our views of the treatment.   The mercurial plan was persisted in for weeks, that the poison of
Venus might without failure be now most thoroughly
driven from its strong holds in the bones and membranes.   Soon after this, he fell into the hands of a
notorious nostrum-vender, who pretended that he never
employed mercury for the cure of any disease.   This
medical adventurer and impostor lured many into his
snares by a vapouring and imposing air and manner.
He not only did not employ mercury to cure diseases,

·but he possessed a secret remedy, he averred, by which he could extract all the mercury deposited by other doctors in the bones of his patients. In a short time he salivated this poor man most violently, and this he accomplished by giving him every night, as I under-·stood, forty-one grains of calomel, twelve grains of rhubarb, and two grains of opium.*

This unfortunate victim of mercury lost a part of his · nose, which sunk in, and most of the palate of his mouth—and continuing under the quack, he at last died of phthisis pulmonalis, as I was informed by a brother of his.

In the summer of 1822, I was called to see a gentle-man affected with a violent attack of the terrific epi-demic, which then desolated the town and neighbour-

---

* The secret composition of this empirical adventurer, which he prescribed, indiscriminately, to cure scrofula, mercurial disease, convulsions, rheumatism, dysentery &c., was made known, to me by a former student of his, now a very correct and respectable phy-sician., This young gentleman, allured by the surreptitious repu-tation of the ready and crafty charlatan, who was then regarded by some of our wiseacres as Æsculapius returned to bless the earth with his profound skill in the treatment of human maladies, com-menced the study of medicine with him; or, rather remained in his shop to be a witness of his miracles in the art of healing all diseases with one remedy. He became disgusted with the ignorant crea-ture's presumption and blustering charlatanry, and abandoned him, though some of the *enlightened* people still adhered to his nostrum-working power. Pearson well remarks, "although there are many who pretend to exclude mercury from their nostrums, yet their perfidious declarations are betrayed by the salivating quality of that mineral, which in defiance of every disguise and combina-tion, will appear to the detection of the impostor."

hood of Louisville.* His constitution was very vigorous; he was a native of the northern part of the United States, and was habitually temperate. He was bled to a large extent a few hours after the accession of the fever, and took a dose of calomel and jalap, which operated slightly. The day after the seizure another physician was called in to attend with me, and it was agreed on in conference to push for mercurialism in the case. He accordingly took ten grains of calomel every four hours, and as his pulse was reduced by the bleeding, no further detraction of blood was practiced. Having been seized with fever the subsequent day myself, the care of the patient was surrendered to the other physician. He continued the calomel, and added inunction. Whilst under this treatment, convulsions came on, the pulse still reduced, the warm bath was employed, and small portions of opium. After my recovery I visited the patient at the request of the third physician, the second one having been attacked with fever. The patient was at this time, fourteen days from the period of the discontinuance of my attendance, affected with mercurial ulcers in the mouth and throat, his discharges were of a tenacious consistence and dark coloured, and he lay in a state of coma. The remedy had not excited ptyalism at all—there being no increased secretion of saliva. The pulse was weak and quick, and the thirst great. The ulcerations came on several days after all remedies were abandoned, and daily grew worse till, apparently, they were extended through the

* For an account of this epidemic fever, see Chapman's Journal, Vol. 8.

intestinal tube, for his anus became ulcerated, and san.
guineous evacuations closed his life.

In the year 1825, a man named Hamilton, was ad.
mitted into the Louisville Marine Hospital, affected
with a very extensive cutaneous disease. Not being in
attendance at the time, I was invited by the attending
physician and surgeon to see the case. It appeared a
matter of much uncertainty with the attending physician and surgeon which of them should conduct the
treatment of the man's case;—they therefore determined
to prescribe for him in consultation. He was a boat-
man, and formerly a British seaman, and in good health
previous to the appearance of the eruption. His general
health was still good. The whole surface of the body
was covered, almost literally, with a furfuracious eruption, which was most crowded on the trunk, before and
behind. When he pulled off his shirt, at our request,
the branny scales fell around him like snow flakes. On his
scrotum, and the inner part of each thigh, in contact
with the scrotum, there were superficial ulcers. The
glans penis was sound, but the inguinal glands were in-
durated and enlarged to a small degree. He told several
different tales, concerning his previous situation, and
thus increased the perplexity of the medical gentlemen,
who sought to ascertain the precise nature of his malady. Some of the physicians and surgeons of the house
who saw the case, considered it lepro vulgaris; while
others regarded it as a good specimen of general herpes.
Several, with myself, in reflecting on the patient's
mode of life, general health, and the character of the
eruption, were convinced that it was syphilitic. To
strengthen the position, which we took, I referred the

15*

gentlemen to the positive declaration of Carmichael, who says, "the true syphilitic eruption is scaly, a circumstance by which it may be distinguished from the eruptions of the other forms of the venereal disease, which we have seen are either papular, pustular, or tubercular.* Candour compels me to state, however, that upon further investigation, I found that this distinguishing criterion, so confidently announced by the eminent surgeon just quoted, is not confided in by very high authority. S. Cooper, in his Surgical Dictionary, makes the following remarks: " There is as little certainty, about the essential characters of a syphilitic eruption, as about the test of every other symptom of the venereal disease, or rather diseases." "It must be allowed," he further observes, " that it is frequently very difficult to say, whether an eruption is syphilitic or not, and an opinion should rather be formed from the history of the case, than from any particular appearance of the eruption itself. Dr. Hennen, in his valuable book, does not pretend to be able to discriminate the true syphilitic eruptions from others, and indeed by what criterion they are to be known, I am myself entirely puzzled to comprehend, after the numerous facts, so fully established by recent experimental inquiries.†

In lepra there is an impairment of general health; and this not being the case with this man, we felt warranted in pronouncing the disease not to be leprous. Herpes is a vesicular affection, and therefore altogether dissimilar to this eruption. Besides, the fellow acknowledged

* Carmichael on Venereal Disease, Emerson's Edition, p. 292.
† 4th London Edition, Art. Venereal Disease.

to the steward of the institution, that he had venereal congress with a courtezan at St. Louis, about three weeks before he perceived the eruption. The surgeon and physician in attendance treated it not as syphilitic, but as a disease "stat nominis umbra." They purged their patient with saline cathartics, and ordered the black wash to be applied to the ulcers. Under this treatment he did not improve, but under a reduced diet and the purgation, grew weak. This method was persevered in for four weeks, at the end of which time, there were several ulcers on the breasts, and the axillary glands were enlarged. In this condition he fell into the hands of the next attending surgeon in course, who being positive of the venereal origin of the affection, determined at once to assail it most heroically. So poured in the mercury with the utmost precipitation, and soon salivated the patient quite to his satisfaction. But instead of improving under this rash mode of giving mercury, Hamilton grew worse—phagadenic ulcers appeared in different parts of his body, his nose ulcerated, and an afflorescence covered his forehead and face. At times a tensive membranous pain was felt over his brows. He was finally cured, after remaining in the hospital nine months, with arsenic, given in conjunction with cicuta, and by dressing his ulcers with weak citron ointment. He left the house in the spring of 1826, but returned in consequence of exposure to a wet, cool atmosphere, which brought back the disease. One of the surgeons employed Swaim's panacea on him, much to the dissatisfaction of the other surgeons and physicians: for to the honour of the most eminent of the faculty in Louisville, they never connive at quackery in any shape, or under any guise. The man finally quit the house without being perfectly cured, and went to New Orleans, where a dry hot summer effected a complete cure of his case. I saw him afterwards perfectly well. In the above case, small doses of corrosive sublimate, with a decoction of sarsaparilla, should have been given for the eradication of the eruption in the first instance; and the mercury should never have been so lavishly employed.

Dr. Chapman has very judiciously remarked that, "no diseases are so unmanageable by constitutional remedies as those of the surface, and particularly of the cuticle. As one cause of failure, in these cases, much may be ascribed to the manner in which mercury is ordinarily prescribed. Eager to attain its effects, it is too much our habit to pour into the system, and hastily to induce salivation, by which the end in view is usually defeated. "My friend," continues the doctor, in a note, "Dr. Holcombe, of New Jersey, has justly acquired much celebrity for his uncommon success in the management of chronic eruptions and obstinate ulcers. He lately assured me, that his practice consists in giving the tenth of a grain of corrosive mercury twice a day for months, and the decoction of dulcamara. By this course, he recently cured a case of prurigo formicans, which had baffled the efforts of some of the best practitioners of this city."*

A man, named Memmer, died from excessive inflammation, terminating in gangrene, of the mouth and throat, several years ago in the Louisville Marine Hos-

* Chapman's Mat. Med. 6th Ed. vol. II. p. 224.

pital. Upon inquiry into the history of the case, it appeared that a drunken doctor at Shippingport, had given him large quantities of calomel for the cure of ague and fever. Memmer had been a patient of mine in the hospital the year before for dyspepsia, of the most aggravated character I ever witnessed; which resulted from his taking, by a physician's directions, in Mississippi, some where, a powerful dose of almost undiluted nitric acid, "to eat off an ulcer he had in his liver," as the sage doctor elegantly described it. From the symptoms present, I fully thought that there existed an ulcer in his stomach. After a tedious confinement, he got well of the dyspepsia. After his death from the excessive mercurial irritation, we carefully examined his stomach, as well as the other organs. No trace of organic lesion could be seen in the stomach, and no globules of mercury could be detected in the salivary glands, or any other part, although some of the physicians present, were firm believers in that dogma.

On the 13th November, 1832, I was requested to meet a very intelligent country practitioner, in a case of some considerable delicacy and interest. The patient was a young married man, a lawyer by profession, who had been confined to his room for several months. The history of the case, as gathered from the attending physician, and the gentleman himself, was the following:— Before marriage, he had contracted a chancre, which was treated with caustic, and a quick and severe mercurialism. The chancre disappeared, and a few months afterwards he entered the matrimonial state. Several months after marriage, upon some exposure, he became affected with sore throat, and ulcerations of the surface

of the body.   A medical man being consulted, looked
upon the symptoms as essentially syphilitic, and put
the patient under the use of blue-pill.   But he grew
worse.   Another physician being sent for, actively de-
pleted him, holding, as he told me in our conference
on the case, the doctrine of Broussais, that there was no
peculiar difference between one inflammation and another, only in the degree of action of the affected parts.
Under the guidance of this very erroneous position, he
had bled his patient several times, and kept him on a
very reduced diet, occasionally exhibiting blue-pill to
act on the liver.   The state of the young gentleman,
when I saw him, was hazardous.   There were ulcers
on his back, breast, arms and legs; his throat was quite
sore, and the glans penis had become ulcerated.   His
wife suffered from no infection.   There was an injunc-
tion to refrain from his marital rights, but it was a matter of doubt whether he obeyed.   In our conversation
on the case, no agreement of opinion, as regarded the
treatment, took place, though the disease was considered by both of us as mercurial.   The medical attendant persisted in his Broussian views, and seemed
resolutely bent on fulfilling the legitimate indications of
treatment, founded on such wrong conceptions of the
nature of inflammation.   The patient died during that
winter.

The following corollaries are fairly deducible from
the reflections and facts presented in the foregoing discussion.

1. That mercury has two modes of action, a local
and general.

2. That mercury operates on the living solids, and does not enter the blood.

3. That there is nothing so specific in the mercurial disease, as should deter us from pursuing a line of practice, built upon our knowledge of inflammation, as modified by texture, the state of the constitution, and the effects of remedies.

4. That to restore the secretions generally, and especially that of the skin, should be our polar star in such cases.

When mercury acts strongly as a local irritant, its agency on the glandular apparatus and capillary system is defeated. Paris, in his excellent work has some judicious suggestions on this point, and he pertinently puts the question, " would it not appear that *powerful doses rather produce a local than general effect.*" He illustrates the operation of medicines given in a large or small dose, by the result of impressions made on the skin—if the impression be violent local pain is induced; but if gentle, a general sensation is excited. But a mercurial medicine, such as calomel, may not only act locally on the stomach, and thus bring on immediate vomiting and purging, in consequence of which local effect, its general alterant impression will be defeated; it may likewise create another kind of local circumscribed irritation, a little farther diffused, which will be entirely subversive of its best constitutional agency—and this irritation may be properly viewed essentially a disease created by the remedy. Alley has seen the hydrargyria, or eczema mercuriale, follow the administration of a few grains of the mildest preparation of mercury, before the mercurial action could have been excited. But this irritation instead of being expended on the skin, may be directed to the mouth, especially in children. It appears to me, that much confusion has existed in the minds of medical men, as regards the efficacy of the mercurial action in fever. Inflammation, and even ulceration, of the mouth may take place without the fever giving away. Here the remedy acts as a local irritant, and will not suppress the febrile movements. But whenever the proper con- stitutional agency of mercury can be secured in fever, the secretions of bile, urine and sweat, are restored by that alterant or modifying influence, and whether you rouse the salivary glands into very exalted action or not, you cure the fever.

Fordyce, in his work on Fever, has made some pro- found reflections in reference to the twofold effects of tartar emetic. When it nauseates in fever, it simply depresses the powers of the system; but given in doses, not to nauseate, it exerts a more favourable impression on the functions, and gently conducts the organs back to their original type of health. Digitalis has a similar mode of operation. Given in such quantity as to sen- sibly affect the stomach, it lowers the heart's action in a powerful manner, but when administered in small doses, it influences the secretory office of the kidneys. The physiological action of mercury, antimony, arsenic and other potent instruments of medical art, may be considered as local and remote. If the local action be very powerful, then we have a case of poisoning—such as may be produced by corrosive sublimate, tartar emetic, &c. If not sufficiently powerful to destroy life in a short time, then other organs are affected. Some poisons affect with a peculiar transference of irritation, one organ or circle of tissues, and leave certain other organs free, comparatively, from their influence. Thus infusion of tobacco, and upas antiar, act, with certain relevancy, on the heart. Mr. Brodie's experiments prove this, for he found that when the infusion of either of these poisons was injected into any part of the body, it speedily caused a cessation of the heart's action, and after death the heart was not irritable to galvanism. Majendie found that in poisoning with tartar emetic, the lungs were inflamed, and sometimes even hapatized.

Nux vomica acts on the spine, and narcotics on the brain. Arsenic, applied to the skin, will inflame the alimentary mucous tissue—cantharides the urinary organs—spurred rye, when used as an article of diet, causes gangrene of the limbs. The effects of a powerful agent, such as mercury, well managed, are exceedingly multifarious. By a variety of causes its action may be, almost in an endless manner, modified. The most important to notice, in a brief way, 1 are quantity—2 chemical preparation—3 combination with other remedies—4 points of the body to which applied—5 age and idiosyncrasy—6 certain states of disease.

I pretend not to penetrate further into the action of mercury on the body, than a careful observation of the phenomena upon its exhibition. No doubt it acts in accordance with the laws of the system—but to endeavour to cover the whole field of the controversy by any cant medical phrase—such as sympathy, or purification of the blood, is in violation of sound philosophy.

16

As " interpreters and ministers of nature," we must
watch her modes of working, and not force her into
any narrow circumscriptions of action.   Nor are we to
substitute 'our fancies for her facts—" imposing gay
deliriums for truths."   We must believe what we can
prove, and leave the rest in doubt and mystery.

The cases given in this essay, exemplify the position
taken.   In the child's case, the operation of the calomel
on the bowels and bilious secretion, was interfered with
by the cold water drank.   It is a well known fact, that
salivation is peculiarly hazardous in children under
eight years of age.   It is impossible to produce it in
very young children, and when mercury makes the
mouth sore in children of a tender age, the salivary
glands are not excited into an increase of secretory
action, but ulceration of the gums and cheeks, and
sometimes the entire destruction of the alveolar process takes place   The gums turn white and recede from
the teeth, which drop out, and mortification, if the disease is severe, soon destroys the cheeks.   Cold drinks
freely indulged in, when the febrile action is not very
high, I consider detrimental, when calomel is taken.
They act injuriously in two ways—first, by exciting
a disturbing action in the stomach, inimical to the
kindly cathartic effect of the medicine; and the second
place, by reducing the functional activity of the der-
moid tissue.   Whatever affects the vital properties and
susceptibilities of the stomach and skin, most interferes
with the regular due exertion of mercury on the system.   To give opium with calomel in fever, is injudicious, unless the powers of life are sunk.   Opium arrests
secretory action in most of the organs, and augments

the local inflammations. Where a stimulus is needed, camphor or Virginia snake-root, in decoction, is preferable to opium. Where pain exists, and it is desirable to tranquilize the patient, then opium must be united with the calomel.

There is nothing peculiar or specific in the inflammation produced by the irritating agency of mercury on the animal economy. Sulphur has been consecrated by the darkened views of humorilism to the cure of mercurial diseases, from the idle and ridiculous supposition that it acted chemically on the mercury floating at large in the blood, and committing sundry depredations. By its effects upon the skin and bowels, sulphur may be of some service in such cases.

Physicians formerly seemed afraid to approach mercurial affection with the ordinary remedies for inflammation, but of late a better practice has obtained. The condition of the system should never be lost sight of in conducting the cure of mercurial affections. In treating severe ptyalism it is sometimes proper to purge with the neutral salts, in order that a revulsive action should be set up. But where the pulse is weak, and the skin below the natural temperature, the warm bath, and Dover's powder are the most eligible remedies. The best local remedy is the sulphate of copper, with bark and charcoal, where ulcers exist in the mouth. The sugar of lead is a most excellent remedy, where the inflammation is intense. It is to be used as a wash for the mouth. Blisters over the enlarged parotid glands are at times demanded. Gentle emetics are often of much advantage, and tart. emetic given in small portions acts very favourably, where there exists much force in the heart and arteries. The state of the skin must be watched, most sedulously watched: a proper degree of functional energy must be maintained in it.

Arsenic exerts a strong action on the skin and subcutaneous cellular tissue, as is evinced in its curing elephantiasis, and in producing effusions about the upper parts of the face. Powdered sarsaparilla, given as Brodie directs, I have used within a year or two with much satisfaction. Upon it and Fowler's solution I mainly rely in mercurial ulcerations of the surface. Sometimes by stimulating these ulcers of the skin and sub-cutaneous cellular tissue, by the following lotion they have been aroused into healthy action, after other dressings had failed.

℞ Sulphas Cupri ℈j
  Balsam Copaivæ ℥ ss
  Pulv. Gum Arabic ℨ ij
  Water ℥ vj
  M.

Or a strong solution of white vitriol, twenty or thirty grains to the ounce of water, will often be of signal efficacy.

In irritable weakened constitutions a mild generous diet must be allowed—even a little wine, or malt liquors, should the patient's strength require either, or his previous habits have rendered such drinks necessary.

A STATEMENT

OF THE CIRCUMSTANCES CONNECTED WITH THE SUDDEN DEATH OF EIGHT PERSONS WHO PARTOOK OF COLD CUSTARD IN LOUISVILLE, KY.

Early in June, 1834, a very great sensation was produced in the city of Louisville by the sudden death of eight individuals belonging to a respectable family of relations and dependents. And as every person who died had partaken of a cold custard, a suspicion was hastily created that they had been poisoned. This suspicion received confirmation from the fact that some negroes belonging to the family, in which the custard was prepared, had been suspected of a robbery committed on the premises several weeks previous to this sad period, and were much exasperated in consequence of the suspicion, and attempts at a discovery of the stolen goods. Arsenic had been inquired for at one of the drug stores of the city by a negro man in the name of the family, in which the deaths occurred. It was refused, and no subsequent call at that drug store was made for it.

Three or four negroes were put in jail upon these grounds of suspicion, and one of the bodies disinterred for examination. I was invited with other physicians to attend the post mortem examination of the disinterred body. Upon my arrival at the house in which the examination of the body was to take place, I found several of our most respectable physicians present. At this meeting, and subsequent to the post mortem inves-

16 *

tigation, a committee of four physicians, then present, was appointed to collect all the facts pertaining to the subject of these sudden deaths, and submit a report of the result of their inquiry at as early a date as possible to a meeting of the faculty, to be called whenever they were ready to communicate that result.   On June 13th nineteen physicians met agreeably to the request of the committee, at which meeting Dr. T. S. Bell, chairman of the committee, read the following report.

" At a meeting of the physicians of Louisville on the 10th inst. it was resolved that ' Drs. Bell, Pendergrast, Salbot, and Wantyn, be appointed a committee to investigate all the circumstances attending the onset, progress and termination of the late cases in the Buckner family, and report the result of their deliberations to the faculty.' "

" The committee appointed under the foregoing resolution, respectfully report, that they have examined with much care, the various statements which have come to them in a tangible form, from sources entitled to attention.   In submitting these facts to your consideration, the committee feel, in the faithful discharge of their duty, bound to abstain from the expression of individual opinion on the facts; their exclusive business is to collect, arrange, and present them, and any argument which they may enter into, will be more for the elucidation of truth, than for the purpose of influencing a particular bias.   Divesting ourselves, as much as possible from the deep and pervading excitement, which is sweeping through this community on the subject, we have endeavoured to guard against the approach of every thing that would prevent a faithful narrative of all the circumstances, placed within our reach.   If the anxieties of the public mind could have slumbered, we might with more time, have presented a more satisfactory report; but so far from diminishing, they are on the increase—rumour, on its busy wings, is afloat, magnifying the slightest incident, into a great one, and giving to its crude fancies, the force, dignity, and solemnity of truth.   The public look up to the medical faculty for information, and is anxiously suspended upon the combined result of our inquiries: and animated with a sense of respect for its feelings, we proceed to a statement of *all* the *facts*, we have been able to receive.   It appears that the first cases of disease occurred in the families of Mr. Fontaine and Col. R. Buckner, in the persons of a young lady, connected with the family of Buckner, and a servant boy of Col. Buckner's.   They were attacked in the morning of Sunday, the 7th inst. (8th.) about the same time of day. Miss Vanasdel, the young lady, complained of slight indisposition immediately after breakfast and vomited some coffee which she drank at breakfast. She said but little about her sickness, until towards about eleven o'clock, when, the symptoms becoming somewhat more urgent, such as increased sickness of the stomach and bilious diarrhæa, she consented to permit a physician to be sent for.   It was accordingly done and he found her on his arrival, about half past 11 o'clock, but slightly indisposed, with what he considered a very mild attack of cholera morbus, for such was the appearance of the disease.   Making a prescription for her, he was summoned to the negro boy of Col. Buckner, and found his system nearly collapsed, and the boy vomiting profusely and purging rice water evacuations. After a vigorous effort on the part of the physician, all endea-

vours at his relief were given up—his case was utterly
hopeless. While engaged with the boy, his partner
was called upon to see Miss Vanasdel—reached her at
half past two, and found her collapsed. A livid circle
surrounded the eye lids, the extremities perfectly cold,
with occasional spasms, though very slight ones, pulse
imperceptible, the face extremely cold and covered
with a profuse clammy sweat. Medicines were administered and other measures ordered for her relief—
another physician was summoned in consultation, and
before his arrival the pulse had resumed a thread-like
expression. In consultation it was agreed that it was a
case of cholera, and such was the general appearance of
the case. She had but three rice water discharges before her collapse, and her and the boy died before 12
o'clock at night.

" A black man, belonging to Col. Buckner, and having
a wife at Mr. Fontaine's, was also attacked very violently with a vomiting and purging of water about the
time Miss Vanasdel was so violently affected. His
spasms were not violent and soon ceased under the same
treatment that had failed in her case, and which had
been found frequently successful in attacks of cholera;
he recovered without the appearance of any of those
effects, seen in the convalescence of cholera cases. At
half past 4 o'clock, P. M. on Sunday the 8th inst. Dr.
Talbot informs the committee, he was called to see Mrs.
Foster; he found her with anxious countenance, eyes
sunken, features contracted, slight lividness of the skin,
particularly immediately below the eyes; learned that
her bowels had been actively operated on for the last
half hour—that she had eaten some dinner, and felt as
well as usual up to the commencement of purging, and

then not sick, as expressed by herself. While in the room she took cramp in one foot, shortly after in the other, and in a very short time vomiting supervened and general cramp of the extremities came on, with great anxiety and tossing, and insatiate thirst. In two and a half hours from the commencement of the attack she was pulseless at the wrist, extremities cold and clammy, lived nine hours after, occasionally conversing rationally with her friends, and calmly expired. On Monday morning (9th inst.) about sunrise, was called to Mr. Foster's little daughter, found her restless, tongue clean, pulse regular, round and rather full, skin in good condition, with frequent rice water evacuations from the bowels; vomiting came on, restlessness and anxiety increased, the skin became pale, assumed a light bluish appearance—throughout great thirst, which increased in intensity, the skin remained warm, though declining in temperature, and the pulse regular until about 4 o'clock, P. M., at which time she took light general spasms, and shortly after expired.

"Monday morning, Mrs. Buckner, the mother of the family, was attacked with vomiting, and bilious discharges. Her family physician reached her immediately after she was taken, but notwithstanding strong and repeated efforts for her relief were made, she died in the course of the evening (afternoon) of Monday. She had rice water discharges towards the termination of the case. Up to within a very few hours of her death, with corrugated hands, she had a full, but powerless pulse, whilst her skin was livid, and cramps were present in the hands and feet.

"At 2 o'clock, Monday morning (9th) the son of Mr. Milton Buckner, was attacked with vomiting and purging, and died during the same morning—which attack was a renewal of one which had taken place on the Saturday previous, but which was then arrested by medicine.

" A black boy of Mrs. Pope's, living with Mr. Fontaine, was taken Sunday night (8th) between 10 and 11 o'clock, with violent vomiting—collapsed at 11, without the rice water purging. It came on after he was collapsed. He complained immediately he was taken, that he was burning up all over. He died Monday morning (9th) after breakfast time.

" This is a full, and it is believed, a faithful sketch of the cases up to the time of death. Examinations of tw of the bodies were made. One on Monday, by an individual member of the committee, who was forced by great press of business to make the examination at the only moment of leisure he obtained, and who in that short interval, endeavoured ineffectually to get the aid of the only physicians he could see. Their engagements prevented them from attending the examination. The other examination was made Tuesday afternoon, (the 10th) in presence of seven of the faculty, on the body of Mrs. Pope's boy, who was buried on Monday morning, and disinterred on that afternoon, just before the post mortem inspection.

" The committee have now discharged their duty by bringing forward the facts of the case. ' The common rumours afloat have not been noticed, because it did not belong to the committee to say any thing about them. Their province was to investigate, and bring forward the facts of the case, independent of their individual opinions. "

After the reading of the above report, it was resolved by the meeting, " that from the facts laid before us by Drs. Bell, Talbot, Pendergrast and Wantyn, that the persons referred to, died of cholera asphyxia; but there is some just grounds for an opinion that, stale or sour custard, did act as an exciting cause in producing derangement of the stomach." The facts in reference to the custard, as stated by several of the physicians, who obtained their information from the family, were these. On Thursday, the 5th of June, a custard had been prepared for a wedding, that night to be celebrated in the house of Mrs. Buckner, one of the persons who died. It was discovered, subsequent to its preparation and cooking, that the custard had been made of milk not entirely fresh, as it had undergone some change; the whey in the composition having separated from the curd in a slight degree. Whereupon it was put aside and not used at the supper table of the nuptials. The next day (Friday the 6th,) it was distributed among the immediate relatives of the family. All those who died, ate of this custard on Friday, and some kept it till Saturday, before entirely using all that was sent them. On Friday, several other persons, besides those who died, had partaken of it; some of these were made sick by it, but a few were not.

In addition to the above enumerated seven individuals, Mrs. Fontaine also was seized with symptoms analogous to those detailed as occurring in the other cases, and died (I think) on the day of the meeting of the physicians to receive the above report. Her illness was, like the others, short and characterized by cramps and collapse of the vital energies. So agitated was she with the awful apprehension of being poisoned, that she told a lady of my acquaintance that were it not for this terrible impression haunting her mind, she would soon be well—"but," says she, "see here how much arsenic there is in me"—pulling some tartar, at the same time, from off her teeth—"how can I live when this is so."

Mrs. Foster, Mrs. Fontaine, and the two Buckners mentioned above, were children of old Mrs. Buckner, at whose house the wedding took place. There was a large quantity of the custard made, and it was sent to the families designated above through a hot sun, in different parts of a small city. It had been kept in a cool cellar, in a tin vessel, previous to its distribution. The post mortem examinations of the two cases noticed, conducted to nothing conclusive, as regards poisoning being the cause of the attacks. The boy's stomach contained a large quantity of calomel, in a state of semi-oxide, but was not at all inflamed; and his bowels were filled with a thick rice water secretion, there being no trace of bile within the intestines. Dr. Bell stated that in the other case there was perforation of the stomach, with strong evidences of vascular fullness, and a spot of gangrene on the villous coat.

The report as first read, was much longer than as given above, and it was curtailed by the meeting, by the exclusion of what was considered irrelevant, or superfluous matter. The following sentences are copied from those parts of it which were rejected.

"On the one hand it is argued, that the cases in their general features, bore the certain and characteristic impress of cholera. The vomiting, purging of rice-water, spasms and length of asphyxiated stage, so universally found in cholera, were in these cases." "Upon investigation of all the circumstances of the question, there is at least a probable ground for the belief, that a deleterious agent has had much to do in the cases. We say only a probable ground for belief, because there is no positive testimony on the subject." And again—

"On the supposition that poison was administered, arsenic was not the poison used."

On a careful analysis of the contents of the two stomachs, obtained by opening of the two negroes, nothing but calomel could be detected. The conclusion to which the meeting came, as regards the origin of these melancholy cases, was by no means satisfactory to the public mind. The impression was general, that the negro slaves had poisoned the family, and whatever absence of proof there was, that any poison was given; and however pointed and cogent the facts were in favour of the opinion at which a majority of the faculty arrived, yet a judicial process must be gone into. Whilst the slaves, suspected of the commission of the act of poisoning, were in jail, Dr. T. S. Bell, over his own signature, published in one of the daily newspapers, his opinion, that these people did not die of cholera, but of some kind of poison. His language in the Louisville Journal, of June 23d, is, in part, as follows, whilst animadverting on the resolution passed by the meeting of physicians.

"It is evident" says the Doctor, "now, that whatever analogy there might have been between cholera and some of the cases, no power on earth can weave these into cases of asphyxia. Speak to a physician of a case of asphyxia with a pulse, and he would laugh

17

at it.   A living dead tree, would be a phrase synony-
mous with it.   What confidence then is to be put in
such a decision, under such circumstances ?   A committee reports, among their facts, two cases with pulse and
warm extremities, and the majority of the faculty, on
this testimony of the committee, resolve that they were
cold and pulseless.   It speaks broadly of the benefit of
a resolution, but is not very creditable to the power of
testimony   Any dogma, no matter how obnoxious to
truth, may be thrown into the form of a resolution; but
it is quite another thing to prove it.''   '' That the cases
were not, cholera, I am firmly convinced—that they
were the effects of poison, I am just as certain.''   Here
is downright positive, bold assumption and dogmatism,
with a vengeance.

Dr. Bell heads his article in the newspaper, ''Health
of Louisville;'' and labours through the whole of it to
prove that no choleric predisposition existed in the
atmosphere, and that therefore the custard must have
played a more important part than a mere excitant to
cholera.   The truth was, that cases of cholera asphyxia
were occurring nearly every day in the city at this very
time; and as a proof, I will merely state, that on the
12th of June, I was called in consultation with Dr.
Rogers to see Mr. Raymond and mother, who both
died that day of the disease, after but a few hours
illness.

In this newspaper article, Dr. Bell says, '' I do not
feel at liberty to say any more about the circumstantial
evidence—though this is the weakest link in the chain.
A wish for justice compels me not to intrude into the
precincts of a judicial examination.''   By a wish for justice, the Dr. means that inasmuch as the slaves were

then in prison, waiting their trial before a court of justice, he did not wish to say any more about it. A love of justice, as well as humanity, if not professional courtesy, should have kept him from such a publication. And did the Doctor detect any poisonous substance in the custard, or in the matter ejected from the stomachs of the patients he attended? Not a particle. And when called before the grand jury, who sat soon after his publication, to make solemn inquest upon the guilt of the slaves, " the weakest link in the chain" of the evidence which the Doctor could adduce, was not corroborated by any stronger links. In other words, no true bill was found, and the slaves were liberated. The palpable violation of consistency in opinion on the part of Dr. Bell, is seen by comparing what he says as chairman of the committee, and what he, without due caution, so boldly and peremptorily decides to be true, in his newspaper article. In the first he admits that the "length of the asphyxiated stage," among the other symptoms, "so universally found in cholera, were in these cases;" in the latter, he avers the contrary, as respects the very same cases. In the one instance, to be sure, he addressed those competent to decide on the question; in the other, the appeal was made to the prejudice and ignorance of persons incompetent to arrive at a just conclusion on such a subject. To the great injury of medical science, and the degradation of the profession in the eyes of the public, are newspaper discussions and controversies on medical topics. Avoiding such a mode of agitating the point, I have written the above statement, with a hope that it may prove useful in putting medical men on their guard against the formation of rash and premature opinions on nice and perplexed questions of toxicology, and to persuade them to weigh well, all the bearings of a controverted point, before they too dogmatically declare their thoughts—especially when such a declaration is calculated only to alarm and distress those personally interested, and to hinder the beneficent operation of public sympathy in favour of those accused of such a vile crime as that of poisoning.

Whatever difficulties may embarrass the solution of a litigated topic, we are never to reject the most rational inference, because we cannot free it of all obscurity, nor are we to pronounce upon a question as if we were gifted, by a special revelation of light, to decide according to the rapid glance of our limited intellectual vision. Let the candid and intelligent reader reflect carefully on the above detailed cases, and compare what Orfila, Paris and Fonblanque, Beck or Christison, has written on the symptoms of poisoning, the rapid access of such symptoms, subsequent to the administration of the noxious substance, with the symptoms in the above cases, and the period after eating the custard in which they arose; and can they do otherwise than acknowledge, Dr. Bell's opinion to the contrary notwithstanding, that these persons did not die of poison. By whatever name he may choose to designate their disease, it is apparent that to live one, two and three days, without any symptoms of poisoning making their appearance, is ample proof, besides the total absence of all positive testimony to prove that poison was administered, that it is a most irrational suspicion that could be grafted on such an airy basis—a basis that melts away at the first touch of calm and sober scrutiny.

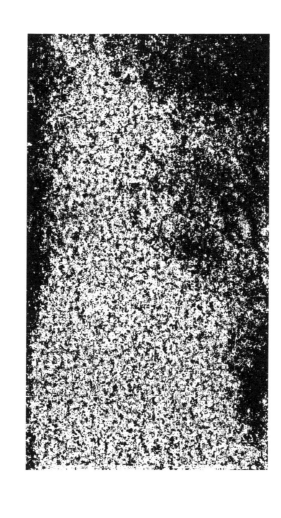

Lightning Source UK Ltd.
Milton Keynes UK
UKHW010757211118
332624UK00007B/337/P